SBAs for the Oral and Maxillofacial Surgery FRCS

SBAs for the Oral and Maxillofacial Surgery FRCS

John Breeze

Consultant Maxillofacial Surgeon, University Hospitals Birmingham NHS Foundation Trust, Senior Lecturer, Imperial College London, UK

Ross Elledge

Consultant Oral and Maxillofacial Surgeon, University Hospitals Birmingham NHS Foundation Trust, UK

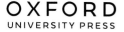

OXFORD
UNIVERSITY PRESS

OXFORD
UNIVERSITY PRESS

Great Clarendon Street, Oxford, OX2 6DP,
United Kingdom

Oxford University Press is a department of the University of Oxford.
It furthers the University's objective of excellence in research, scholarship,
and education by publishing worldwide. Oxford is a registered trade mark of
Oxford University Press in the UK and in certain other countries

© Oxford University Press 2022

The moral rights of the authors have been asserted

First Edition published in 2022

Impression: 1

Published in the United States of America by Oxford University Press
198 Madison Avenue, New York, NY 10016, United States of America

British Library Cataloguing in Publication Data

Data available

Library of Congress Control Number: 2022930321

ISBN 978–0–19–286465–9

DOI: 10.1093/med/9780192864659.001.0001

Printed in the UK by
Bell & Bain Ltd., Glasgow

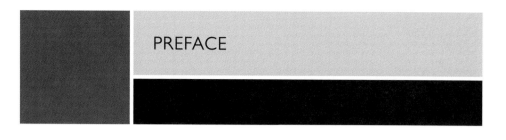

PREFACE

About the examination

The FRCS (OMFS) 'exit' examination is the final assessment of your surgical training and should be seen as a time to demonstrate to your potential peers what you have learned through all those years of study, and that you have the knowledge to act as a consultant. By this point the pressure on you will be immense and the role of this book is to provide candidates with some structure in answering the single-best-answer (SBA) component of the examination. From 2021 it comprises two SBA papers undertaken on a single day. Each paper comprises 120 questions, for which 2 hours 15 minutes is given. The format of the FRCS examination is described on the Joint Committee on Intercollegiate Examinations website (2022).

About this book

This book comprises 300 SBA questions. The questions asked reflect the curriculum for the FRCS examination and will be broken down into key topics. These topics will be weighted according to their relevance in the most recent examinations. The structure of the questions is generally to present you with a clinical scenario and explore how you would manage the situation. The emphasis is very much on what *you* would do, and why, and not just a regurgitation of the latest systematic review. It is therefore somewhat different to any examination you are likely to have sat before, and the authors highly recommend that you find a study partner(s) for this final hurdle. You can only really practise discussing controversial issues and learn how to rationally argue your point by practising this. Your study partner will be your sounding board and support and will likely end up being one of your friends for life; certainly, you are likely to spend more time with them leading up to the examination than anyone else, and so choose carefully.

There has not been another book of its sort for this examination and therefore to a degree this is a work in progress. The editors very much welcome suggestions and improvements for the scenarios, which we would hope to incorporate in future versions. Keep your head high, try not to let the examination affect your day-to-day job, and remember that however much you are suffering, your friends and family are likely to be feeling the pressure as much as you are.

Reference

Joint Committee on Intercollegiate Examinations (2022). Specialities. Oral & Maxillofacial Surgery. Edinburgh: JCIE. https://www.jcie.org.uk/content/content.aspx?id=16 (accessed 28 July 2021).

ACKNOWLEDGEMENTS

Both authors would like to thank Miss Eiling Wu for providing a trainee perspective of many of the questions in this book, and tirelessly reviewing the questions for quality control. We would like to thank Mr Kevin McMillan for providing images 10.4 and 10.6.

John Breeze would like to thank his loving family for the support they have given him when military, clinical, and academic commitments have kept him away from them.

Ross Elledge would like to express gratitude to Sat Parmar for his friendship and support in good times and bad. To his colleagues in the TMJ service in Birmingham (Jason Green and Alan Attard) he gives his continued thanks. Whilst he one day hopes to be their equal, for the time being he regards himself as a contented mentee. He would also like to thank the entire Dermatology team at Solihull Hospital who are the other half of his professional family. The continued support from his academic family at the University of Birmingham, in particular Kirsty Hill and Thomas Addison, cannot go without mention. Finally, he dedicates this book to his children Miles and Sienna, who continue to teach him a better way of looking at the world.

CONTENTS

ABBREVIATIONS

18F–NaF	18F–sodium fluoride
2D	two-dimensional
3D	three-dimensional
5-FU	5-fluorouracil
99mTc	technetium-99m
AAOMS	American Association of Oral and Maxillofacial Surgeons
ACE	angiotensin converting enzyme
ACR	American College of Rheumatology
ADAS	adipocyte-derived adult stem
AFX	atypical fibroxanthoma
AIDS	acquired immunodeficiency syndrome
AJCC	American Joint Committee on Cancer
ANUG	acute necrotizing ulcerative gingivitis
AOB	anterior open bite
ASA	American Society of Anesthesiologists
ATLS	advanced trauma life support
AVM	arteriovenous malformation
BATS	British Association of TMJ Surgeons
BCC	basal cell carcinoma
BFP	buccal fat pad
BSDS	British Society for Dermatological Survey
BSOM	British Society of Oral Medicine
BSSO	bilateral sagittal split osteotomy
C	cervical
CBCT	cone beam computed tomography
CBT	cognitive behavioural therapy
CFM	craniofacial microsomia
CFNG	cross-facial nerve graft
CLND	completion lymph node dissection

CO_2	carbon dioxide
CRP	C-reactive protein
CT	computed tomography
DCIA	distal circumflex iliac artery
DFSP	dermatofibrosarcoma protuberans
DNA	deoxyribonucleic acid
DSO	diffuse sclerosing osteomyelitis
EBV	Epstein–Barr virus
ECD	extracapsular dissection
ECG	electrocardiogram
ELISA	enzyme-linked immunosorbent assay
EMG	electromyography
EMI	Extended Matching Item
END	elective neck dissection
Er:YAG	erbium:yttrium-aluminium-garnet
ESR	erythrocyte sedimentation rate
EULAR	European Alliance of Associations for Rheumatology
FAMM	facial artery musculomucosal
FDA	Food and Drug Administration
FDG	fluorodeoxyglucose
FEH	focal epithelial hyperplasia
FNA	fine needle aspiration
FNAC	fine needle aspiration cytology
FOV	field of view
FRCS (OMFS)	Fellowship of the Royal College of Surgeons in Oral & Maxillofacial Surgery
GIC	glass ionomer cement
GMC	General Medical Council
Gy	Gray
HE	hemimandibular elongation
HH	hemimandibular hyperplasia
HIV	human immunodeficiency virus
HNSCC	head and neck squamous cell carcinoma
HPV	human papillomavirus
HU	Hounsfield units
ICP	intracranial pressure
IgA	immunoglobulin A
IGF-1	insulin-like growth factor 1
IgG4	immunoglobulin G4

IHD	ischaemic heart disease
IMF	intermaxillary fixation
IMRT	intensity-modulated radiation therapy
IOFTN	Index of Orthognathic Functional Treatment Need
IPEH	intravascular papillary endothelial hyperplasia
ISSVA	International Society for the Study of Vascular Anomalies
ITC	isolated tumour cells
IV	intravenous
KFI	Key-Features Item
LAFH	lower anterior face height
LMA	laryngeal mask airway
LMWH	low molecular weight heparin
LRINEC	Laboratory Risk Indicator for Necrotizing Fasciitis
MACH-NC	Meta-analysis of Chemotherapy in Head and Neck Cancer
MACS	minimal access cranial suspension
MALT	mucosa-associated lymphoid tissue
MCQ	multiple choice question
MDCT	multidetector helical computed tomography
MDT	multidisciplinary team
MHRA	Medicines and Healthcare products Regulatory Agency
MMA	maxillomandibular advancement
MMS	Mohs micrographic surgery
MR	magnetic resonance
MRI	magnetic resonance imaging
MRONJ	medication-related osteonecrosis of the jaw
MTA	mineral trioxide aggregate
NG	nasogastric
NHS	National Health Service
NICE	National Institute for Health and Care Excellence
NOAC	non-vitamin K antagonist oral anticoagulant
NOE	naso-orbitoethmoid
NPA	nasopharyngeal airway
NSLN	non-sentinel lymph node
OLP	oral lichen planus
ONF	oronasal fistula
OPG	orthopantomogram
ORIF	open reduction internal fixation
ORN	osteoradionecrosis

OSA	obstructive sleep apnoea
OSCC	oral squamous cell carcinoma
PCR	polymerase chain reaction
PDS	pleomorphic dermal sarcoma
PEEK	polyether ether ketone
PEG	percutaneous endoscopic gastrostomy
PENTOCLO	pentoxifylline, tocopherol, and clodronate
PET	positron emission tomography
PIFP	persistent idiopathic facial pain
PMMA	polymethyl methacrylate
PMMC	pectoralis major myocutaneous
PMSO	posterior maxillary segmental osteotomy
pN+	positive ipsilateral neck nodes
PPP	platelet poor plasma
PPS	parapharyngeal space
QoL	quality of life
RT	radiotherapy
SALT	speech and language therapy
SARME	surgically assisted rapid maxillary expansion
SARPE	surgically assisted rapid palatal expansion
SBA	single best answer
SCC	squamous cell carcinoma
SCI	Script Concordance Item
SLNB	sentinel lymph node biopsy
SMAS	subcutaneous musculoaponeurotic system
SMAS	superficial musculoaponeurotic system
SND	selective neck dissection
SOF	superior orbital fissure
SPECT	single-photon emission computed tomography
SSI	surgical site infection
SSMDT	specialist skin cancer multidisciplinary team
STIR	short tau inversion recovery
STS	sodium tetradecyl sulphate
SUNCT	short-lasting unilateral neuralgiform headache with conjunctival injection and tearing
TAD	temporary anchorage device
TAFH	total anterior face height
TFL	tensor fascia lata
TJR	total joint replacement
TMJ	temporomandibular joint

TNF	tumour necrosis factor
TROG	Trans Tasman Radiation Oncology Group
UPPP	uvulopalatopharyngoplasty
US	ultrasound
VAS	visual analogue scale
VEGF-A	antivascular endothelial growth factor
VP	velopharyngeal
VPD	velopharyngeal dysfunction
VSP	virtual surgical planning
VSSO	vertical subsigmoid osteotomy
WBC	white blood cell
WHO	World Health Organization

The syllabus for the FRCS OMFS exam is vast and will always be challenging for a candidate to cover in its entirety, requiring both breadth and depth of study. The official syllabus was updated in 2021 (Intercollegiate Surgical Curriculum Programme 2021), providing greater clarity. The syllabus is arranged into 12 modules, with topics reflecting the presenting conditions of patients in relation to the specialty. Trainees are expected to have exposure to all topics in phase 2 of training. However, with 300 SBAs asked over both papers it can be daunting to know how to optimize your study. The key is to approach it systematically, and we provide below what we think is a starting block in terms of subjects and consensus papers. The questions have evolved more recently to become more clinically relevant and should be based upon short clinical scenarios or situations you would be faced with as a year-one consultant. The lists below are not exhaustive and will evolve we hope with future iterations of this book. If you are in doubt, the excellent book by Carrie Newlands and Cryus Kerawala will give you an excellent foundation for every topic (Newlands and Kerawala 2020).

References

Intercollegiate Surgical Curriculum Programme (2021). Oral & Maxillofacial Surgery. London: ISCP. https://www.gmc-uk.org/-/media/documents/omfs_inc._trauma_tig.pdf_72601045.pdf (accessed 1 July 2021).

Newlands C, Kerawala C (eds) (2020). *Oral and Maxillofacial Surgery*, 3rd edition. *Oxford Specialist Handbooks in Surgery*. Oxford: Oxford University Press.

Head and Neck Surgical Oncology

Topics

Assessment	Imaging	Types	Surgical treatment	Radiotherapy	Chemotherapy	Outcomes
Two-week pathway Staging (including stage 0) Unknown primary Thyroid staging Histology	PET CT MRI Ultrasound	Oral (including lip) Oropharyngeal Thyroid Paranasal sinuses + nose Miscellaneous (sarcoma)	Margins Thyroid surgery Types of neck dissection Complications (chyle leak) Laryngectomy	Radiotherapy types (e.g. fractionation) Effects of radiotherapy Radiotherapy with implants Indications for radiotherapy	Types, biologics Effects of chemotherapy Indications for chemotherapy	Survival Recurrence Role of HPV Quality of life (QoL)

Recommended reading

Bernier J, Cooper JS, Pajek TF, et al. (2005). Defining risk levels in locally advanced head and neck cancers: a comparative analysis of concurrent postoperative radiation plus chemotherapy trials of the EORTC (#22931) and RTOG (#9501). *Head Neck* **27**(10):843–850.

Bonner JA, Harari PM, Giralt J, et al. (2010). Radiotherapy plus cetuximab for locoregionally advanced head and neck cancer: 5-year survival data from a phase 3 randomised trial and relation between cetuximab-induced rash and survival. *Lancet Oncol* **11**:21–28.

British Association of Head & Neck Oncologists (2020). BAHNO Standards 2020. Petersfield: BAHNO. https://bahno.org.uk/_userfiles/pages/files/final_bahno_standards_2020.pdf.

Brown LS, Lewis-Jones H (2001). Evidence for imaging the mandible in the management of oral squamous cell carcinoma: a review. *Br J Oral Maxillofac Surg* **39**:411–418.

Lassen P, Primdahl H, Johansen J, et al. (2014). Impact of HPV-associated p16-expression on radiotherapy outcome in advanced oropharynx and non-oropharynx cancer. *Radiother Oncol* **113**(3):310–316.

Mehanna H, Wai-Lup W, McConkey CC, et al. (2016). PET-CT surveillance versus neck dissection in advanced head and neck cancer. *N Engl J Med* **374**(15):1444–1454.

Paleri V, Roland N (2015). Head and Neck Cancer: United Kingdom National Multidisciplinary Guidelines. *Journal of Laryngology & Otology* 130(S2). https://www.entuk.org/sites/default/files/files/5th%20edition%20head%20and%20neck%20cancer%20multidisciplinary%20management%20guidelines.pdf.

Schilling C, Stoeckli SJ, Haerle SK, et al. (2015). Sentinel European Node Trial (SENT): 3-year results of sentinel node biopsy in oral cancer. *Eur J Cancer* **51**(18):2777–2784.

Shah J, Patel S, Singh B, Wong R (2019). *Jatin Shah's Head and Neck Surgery and Oncology*, 5th edition. Philadelphia: Elsevier.

Shaw RJ, Brown JS, Wodger JA, et al. (2004). The influence of the pattern of mandibular invasion on recurrence and survival in oral squamous cell carcinoma. *Head Neck* **26**(10):861–869.

Questions in this book

1. Types of radiotherapy.
2. Neck dissections.
3. Complications of radiotherapy.
4. Staging of paranasal sinus cancer.
5. American Joint Committee on Cancer (AJCC) staging of cancer.
6. Treatment of squamous cell carcinoma of the lip.
7. Split skin grafts.
8. 'Cannot intubate cannot ventilate' scenario.
9. Intensity-modulated radiation therapy (IMRT) radiotherapy.
10. Pre-operative patient optimization.
11. Thyroid cancer staging.
12. Oropharyngeal squamous cell carcinoma.
13. Thyroid lesions.
14. Chemotherapy.
15. Chemotherapy.
16. The unknown primary.

17. Tumour site imaging.
18. Mandible metastasis.
19. Quality of life.
20. Pathology of oral cancer.
21. Laryngeal cancer.
22. Sentinel node biopsy.
23. Indications for radiotherapy.
24. Recurrence.
25. The N + neck.
26. The unknown primary.
27. Lymph node levels and boundaries.
28. Palliation in cancer.
29. Core biopsy.
30. Speech and swallowing.

Orthognathic Surgery

Topics

Assessment	Planning	Perisurgical orthodontics	Maxilla surgery	Mandible surgery	Other
History Examination Imaging including SPECT Diagnosis Role of TMJ disorders	Cephalometrics Model surgery Virtual surgical planning (2D and 3D) Aesthetics	Concepts Pre-surgical Functional appliances Post-surgical	Le Fort I Variations SARPE Soft tissue changes Le Fort II and modifications Segmental	BSSO including modifications Vertical osteotomies and modifications Segmental	Genioplasty Bone grafting Implants Stability Distraction Obstructive sleep apnoea Complications

Recommended reading

Brennan PA, Schliephake H, Ghali GE, Cascarini L (2007). *Maxillofacial Surgery*, 3rd edition. London: Churchill Livingstone.

Harris M, Hunt N (2008). *Fundamentals of Orthognathic Surgery*, 2nd edition. London: Imperial College Press.

Ireland AJ, Cunningham SJ, Petrie A, et al. (2014). An Index of Orthognathic Functional Treatment Need (IOFTN). *J Orthodont* **41**:77–83.

Jedrzejewski M, Smektala T, Sporniak-Tutak K, Olszewski R (2015). Pre-operative, intra-operative, and post-operative complications in orthognathic surgery: a systematic review. *Clin Oral Invest* **19**:969–977.

Posnick JC (2014). *Orthognathic Surgery: Principles and Practice*. St Louis: Elsevier.

Reyneke JP, Ferretti C (2007). Anterior open bite correction by Le Fort I or bilateral sagittal split osteotomy. *Oral Maxillofac Surg Clin N Am* **19**:321–338.

Sansaer K, Raghav M, Mallya SM, Karjodkar F (2015). Management-related outcomes and radiographic findings of idiopathic condylar resorption: a systematic review. *Int J Oral Maxillofac Surg* **44**:209–216.

Questions in this book

1. Condylar hyperplasia.
2. Bone graft platelet-rich plasma.
3. Radiation doses.
4. Crouzon's sleep apnoea.
5. Mandibular midline distraction.
6. Posterior maxillary segmental osteotomy.
7. Blood supply maxilla.
8. Maxillary midline distraction
9. Role of PET–CT scanning.
10. Hemimandibular hyperplasia.
11. Stepped Le Fort I osteotomy.
12. Reduction glossectomy.
13. Index of orthodontic treatment need.
14. Hemimandibular elongation.
15. Vertical subsigmoid osteotomy.
16. Ankylosing spondylitis.
17. Pre-operative TMJ symptoms.
18. Obstructive sleep apnoea.
19. Antibiotics for post-operative infection.
20. Anterior open bite.
21. Segmental osteotomies.
22. Soft tissue movements following osteotomy.
23. Kohle osteotomy.
24. Cranial nerve palsies following osteotomy.
25. Class 2 skeletal relationship.

Skin Surgery

Topics

Assessment	Types	Surgical treatment	Non-surgical treatment	Miscellaneous
History	BCC	Excision margins	Radiotherapy	Perioperative care
Examination	SCC	Management of regional	Chemotherapy	including anticoagulants
Imaging	Melanoma	metastases	Biologic agents	Wound care and
Staging	Adnexal	Mohs micrographic surgery	Cryotherapy	dressings
Sentinel lymph		Recurrence		
node biopsy		Surgical techniques		

Recommended reading

Betti R, Menni S, Radaelli G, et al. (2010). Micronodular basal cell carcinoma: a distinct subtype? Relationship with nodular and infiltrative basal cell carcinomas. *J Dermatol* **37**:611–616.

British Association of Dermatologists (undated). Clinical Guidelines. London: BAD. https://www.bad.org.uk/healthcare-professionals/clinical-standards/clinical-guidelines.

Faries MB, Thompson JF, Cochran RH, et al. (2017). Completion dissection or observation for sentinel node metastasis in melanoma. *N Engl J Med* **376**(23):2211–2222.

Green B, Godden D, Brennan PA (2015). Malignant cutaneous adnexal tumours of the head and neck: an update on management. *Br J Oral Maxillofac Surg* **53**:485–490.

Gurney B, Newlands C (2014). Management of regional metastatic disease in head and neck cutaneous malignancy. 1. Cutaneous squamous cell carcinoma. *Br J Oral Maxillofac Surg* **52**:294–300.

Janis J (2014). *Essentials of Plastic Surgery*, 2nd edition. Boca Raton: CRC Press.

Keohane SG, Botting J, Budny PG, et al. (2021). British Association of Dermatologists guidelines for the management of people with cutaneous squamous cell carcinoma 2020. *Br J Dermatol* **184**:401–414.

Marsden JR, Newton-Bishop JA, Burrows L, et al. (2010). Revised UK guidelines for the management of cutaneous melanoma *Br J Dermatol* **163**:238–256.

Morton DL, Thompson JF, Cochran AJ, et al. (2014). Final trial report of sentinel node biopsy versus nodal observation in melanoma. *N Engl J Med* **370**(7):599–609.

Newlands C, Gurney B (2014). Management of regional metastatic disease in head and neck cutaneous malignancy. 2. Cutaneous malignant melanoma. *Br J Oral Maxillofac Surg* **52**:301–307.

Pavri SN, Clune J, Ariyan S, Narayan D (2016). Malignant melanoma: beyond the basics. *Plast Recon Surg J* **138**(2):330e–340e.

Telfer NR, Colver GB, Morton CA. (2008). Guidelines for the management of basal cell carcinoma *Br J Dermatol* **159**:35–48.

Van der Ploeg APT, van Akkooi ACJ, Rutkowski PR, et al. (2011). Prognosis in patients with sentinel node-positive melanoma is accurately defined by the combined Rotterdam tumour load and Dewar topography criteria. *J Clin Oncol* **29**(16):2206–2214.

Questions in this book

1. Basal cell carcinoma margins.
2. Squamous cell carcinoma margins.
3. Pigmented lesions.
4. Breslow thickness.
5. Basal cell carcinoma treatment types.
6. Basal cell carcinoma treatment types.
7. Squamous cell carcinoma treatment types.
8. Squamous cell carcinoma treatment types.
9. Fitness for skin cancer surgery.
10. Assessment of a skin lesion.
11. Mohs micrographic surgery.
12. Melanoma.
13. Sentinel lymph node biopsy.
14. Skin grafts.
15. Lentigo melanoma.
16. Infiltrative basal cell carcinoma.
17. Mohs micrographic surgery.
18. Z-plasty.
19. Basal cell carcinoma re-excision.
20. Basal cell carcinoma treatment types.

21. Skin anatomy.
22. Reconstruction techniques.
23. Suturing techniques.
24. Dermoscopy.
25. Cryosurgery.

Head and Neck Trauma Surgery

Topics

Assessment	Major trauma	Anatomical areas	Surgery	Fixation principles	Additional
History	Principles	Mandible	Closed	Plates and screws	Intraoperative
Examination	Assessment	Maxilla	Open +/	Osteosynthesis	guidance
Imaging	ATLS	Nose	– reduction	types	Intraoperative CT
Classifications	Transfusion	NOE	Maxillary	Champey	Concomitant
(including neck)	protocols	Orbit	mandibular	Conservative	injuries
Visual	Trauma	Frontal	fixation	management	Head injury
Nasolacrimal	centres	Zygoma	External fixators		
Virtual surgical		Dentoalveolar	Surgical		
planning		Base of skull	approaches		
Follow-up		Panfacial	Sequencing		
Medicolegal		Penetrating	Complications		
		neck injury	Late repair		
		Soft tissue injury			

Recommended reading

Abdel-Galil K, Loukota R (2010). Fractures of the mandibular condyle: evidence base and current concepts of management. *Br J Oral Maxillofac Surg* **48**:520–526.

Ehrenfeld M, Neal Futran N, Manson P, Prein J (2020). *Advanced Craniomaxillofacial Surgery. Tumor, Corrective Bone Surgery and Trauma.* Davos: AO Foundation.

Ellis III E, Zide MF (2019). *Surgical Approaches to the Facial Skeleton*, 3rd edition. Philadelphia: Wolters Kluwer.

Ellis III E, Figari M, Shimozato K, Sánchez Aniceto G (undated). CMF Online Surgery Reference Guide. Davos: AO Foundation. https://surgeryreference.aofoundation.org/cmf/trauma.

Evans BT, Webb AAC. (2007). Post-traumatic orbital reconstruction: anatomical landmarks and the concept of the deep orbit. *Br J Oral Maxillofac Surg* **45**:183–189.

Jaquiery C, Aeppli C, Cornelius P, et al. (2007). Reconstruction of orbital wall defects: critical review of 72 patients. *Int J Oral Maxillofac Surg* **36**:193–199.

Perry M (2009). Maxillofacial trauma—developments, innovations and controversies. *Injury* **40**:1252–1259.

Perry M, Holmes S (2014). *Atlas of Operative Maxillofacial Trauma Surgery: Primary Repair of Facial Injuries.* London: Springer.

Questions in this book

1. Fascial space infections.
2. Penetrating neck injury.

3. Coronoid fractures.
4. Open reduction and internal fixation of the condyle.
5. Nasal septal haematoma.
6. Third molar fracture line.
7. Orbital floor fracture.
8. Orbital floor fracture.
9. Naso-orbital-ethmoidal fracture assessment.
10. Mandible fracture complications
11. Orbital roof fracture.
12. Mandible fracture in a child.
13. Scars following facial lacerations.
14. Orbital floor fracture.
15. Use of lag screws.
16. Dog bites.
17. Treatment of frontal sinus indentation.
18. Marginal mandibular nerve damage.
19. Facial nerve weakness.
20. Blood loss.
21. Sialocele.
22. Decompressive craniectomy.
23. Submental intubation.
24. Topical negative pressure therapy.
25. Orbital assessment.
26. Zygoma fracture.
27. Abscess following a condyle fracture.
28. Penetrating neck injury.
29. Wound dehiscence.
30. Suturing techniques.

Salivary Gland Surgery

Topics

Assessment	Malignancy	Benign lesions	Treatment	Others
History	Subtypes	Tumours	Parotidectomy—types,	Xerostomia
Examination	Grading	Stones	complications, ECD	Localized gland swelling
MRI	Staging	Strictures	Submandibular glans excision	Diffuse gland swelling
Ultrasound	Neck dissection	Ranula	Sublingual gland excision	Physiology of glands
CT	Adjuvant treatment		Interventional radiology	Sjögren's
Sialography	Recurrence		techniques (dilatation, basket)	Infection including
Sialendoscopy	Follow-up		Endoscopic techniques	microbiology
Anatomy			Lithotripsy	Autoimmune

Recommended reading

Atienza G, Lopez-Cedrun JL (2015). Management of obstructive salivary disorders by sialendoscopy: a systematic review. *Br J Oral Maxillofac Surg* **53**:507–519.

Burke CJ, Thomas RH, Howlett D (2011). Imaging the major salivary glands. *Br J Oral Maxillofac Surg* **49**:261–269.

Howlett DC, Skelton E, Moody AB (2015). Establishing an accurate diagnosis of a parotid lump: evaluation of the current biopsy methods—fine needle aspiration cytology, ultrasound-guided core biopsy and intraoperative frozen section. *Br J Oral Maxillofac Surg* **53**:580–583.

McGurk M, Combes J (eds) (2012). *Controversies in the Management of Salivary Gland Disease*, 2nd edition. Oxford: Oxford University Press.

McGurk M, Makdissi J, Brown JE (2004). Intra-oral removal of stones from the hilum of the submandibular gland: report of technique and morbidity. *Int J Oral Maxillofac Surg* **33**:683–686.

Renehan AG, Gleave EN, Slevin NJ, McGurk M (1999). Clinico-pathological and treatment-related factors influencing survival in parotid cancer. *Br J Cancer* **80**(8):1296–1300.

Terhaard CH, Lubsen H, Van der Tweel I, et al. (2004). Salivary gland carcinoma: independent prognostic factors for locoregional control, distant metastases and overall survival: results of the Dutch head and neck oncology cooperative group. *Head Neck* **26**(8):692–693.

Terhaard CHJ, Lubsen H, Rasche CRN, et al. (2005). The role of radiotherapy in the treatment of malignant salivary gland tumours. *Head Neck* **61**(1):103–111.

Van der Poorten VLM, Balm AJM, Hilgers FJM (2002). Management of cancer of the parotid gland. *Curr Opin Otolaryngol Head Neck Surg* **10**:134–144.

Questions in this book

1. Warthin's tumour.
2. Sialithiasis.
3. Basal cell adenoma.
4. Sjögren's syndrome.
5. Adjuvant radiotherapy.
6. Sjögren's syndrome.
7. Sjögren's syndrome.
8. Mikulicz's disease.
9. Frey's syndrome.
10. Ranula.
11. Mucosa-associated lymphoid tissue (MALT) lymphoma.
12. Primary SCC parotid.
13. Extracorporeal lithotripsy.
14. Pre-styloid parapharyngeal space.
15. Management of recurrence.

Temperomandibular Joint Disorders

Topics

Assessment	Conditions	Surgery	Non-surgical treatment
History	Meniscal disease	Open arthroplasty	Botulinum toxin
Examination	Osteoarthritis	Eminectomy	Medical therapy
Anatomy	Ankylosis	Autologous joint replacement	Splint therapy
Plain imaging	Myofascial pain	Meniscopexy	
CT	Dislocation	Alloplastic joint replacement	
MRI	Autoimmune	and indications	
Arthroscopy	Trismus	Complications	
Wilkes classification	Septic arthritis		
Follow-up	Neoplasia (benign, malignant)		
	Idiopathic condylar resorption		

Recommended reading

Ahmed N, Sidebottom A (2012). The role of arthroscopy and arthrocentesis in TMJ management. *Face Mouth Jaw Surg* **2**(1):22–28.

Idle M, Monaghan A (2016). *Challenging Concepts in Oral and Maxillofacial Surgery: Cases with Expert Commentary Paperback*. Oxford: Oxford University Press.

Kaban LB, Bouchard C, Troulis MJ (2009). A protocol for management of temporomandibular joint ankylosis in children. *J Oral Maxilllofac Surg* **67**:1966–1978.

Mercuri LG (2016). *Temporomandibular Joint Total Joint Replacement—TMJ TJR*. Cham: Springer.

National Institute for Health and Clinical Excellence (2014). Total prosthetic replacement of the temporomandibular joint. Interventional procedures guidance [IPG500]. London: NICE. https://www.nice.org.uk/guidance/ipg500.

Sidebottom AJ (2008). Guidelines for the replacement of temporomandibular joints in the United Kingdom. *Br J Oral Maxillofac Surg* **46**:146–147.

Sidebottom AJ (2009). Current thinking in temporomandibular joint management. *Br J Oral Maxillofac Surg* **47**:91–94.

Stonehouse-Smith D, Begley A, Dodd M (2020). Clinical evaluation of botulinum toxin A in the management of temporomandibular myofascial pain. *Br J Oral Maxillofac Surg* **58**:190–193.

Questions in this book

1. Joint dislocation.
2. Treatment options for surgery.
3. Imaging of the joint.
4. Joint ankylosis
5. Laxity conditions.
6. Imaging of the joint.
7. Arthritis.
8. Botulinum toxin.
9. Botulinum toxin.
10. Chondrosarcoma.

11. Joint replacement.

12. Fracture dislocation.

13. Interposition arthroplasty materials.

14. Joint replacement.

15. Metal hypersensitivity.

Bone Disease

Topics

Osteonecrosis	Benign tumours	Malignant	Cysts	Fibro osseous	Other
Osteoradionecrosis MRONJ	Ameloblastoma Odontogenic keratocyst Giant cell lesions	Primary bone tumours Secondary deposits Myeloma Osteosarcoma	Radicular Dentigerous Residual Periodontal Aneurysmal	Fibrous dysplasia Fibro osseous dysplasia Cementoma Giant cell lesions including cherubism Fibro osseous neoplasms	Osteomyelitis Eosinophilic granuloma Garre's Odontomes Paget's Osteosclerosis Renal osteodystrophy

Recommended reading

Chrcanovic BR, Gomez RS (2017). Recurrence probability for keratocystic odontogenic tumours: an analysis of 6427 cases. *J Craniomaxillofac Surg* **45**:244–251.

Kaczmarzyk T, Mojsa I, Stypulkowska J (2012). A systematic review of the recurrence rate for keratocystic odontogenic tumour in relation to treatment modalities. *Int J Oral Maxillofac Surg* **41**:756–767.

McLeod NMH, Patel V, Kusanale A, et al. (2011). Bisphosphonate osteonecrosis of the jaw: a literature review of UK policies versus international policies on the management of bisphosphonate osteonecrosis of the jaw. *Br J Oral Maxillofac Surg* **49**:335–342.

Parmar S, al-Qamachi L, Aga H (2016). Ameloblastomas of the mandible and maxilla. *Curr Opin Otolaryngol Head Neck Surg* **24**:148–154.

Pogrel AM (2012). The diagnosis and management of giant cell lesions of the jaws. *Annals Maxillofac Surg* **2**(2):102–106.

Ruggiero SL, Dodson TB, Fantasia J, et al. (2014). American Association of Oral and Maxillofacial Surgeons position paper on medication-related osteonecrosis of the jaw—2014 update. *J Oral Maxillofac Surg* 72(10):1938–1956.

Questions in this book

1. Medication-related osteonecrosis of the jaws.

2. Unicystic ameloblastoma.

3. Odontogenic keratocyst.

4. Odontogenic keratocyst.

5. Osteomyelitis.
6. Odontome.
7. Central giant cell granuloma.
8. Medication-related osteonecrosis of the jaws.
9. Osteomyelitis.
10. Unicystic ameloblastoma.
11. Myeloma mandible.
12. Odontogenic keratocyst.
13. Eosinophilic granuloma.
14. Giant cell granuloma histology.
15. Dentigerous cyst.

Oral Medicine

Topics

Swellings	Ulcers	Blisters	Red and white patches	Pigmentation	Pain	Other
Wegener's	Recurrent	Pemphigus	Potentially	Melanocytic naevus	Trigeminal	Mucosal histology
Tongue swelling	Aphthous	Pemphigoid	malignant	Melanoma	neuralgia	Cytology
Orofacial	ulceration	Immunofluorescence	conditions versus	Peutz–Jeghers	Migraine	Swabs and smears
granulomatosis	Behçet's	Desquamative	lesions	Addison's	Temporal	Drugs
Crohn's	Epstein–Barr	gingivitis	Dysplasia	Kaposi	arteritis	Steroids
Pyogenic	Herpangina	Erythema multiforme	Lichen planus	Hereditary	Atypical	Langerhans cell
granuloma	ANUG	Herpes simplex	Leukoplakia	telangectasia	facial pain	histiocytosis
Papilloma	Noma	Herpes zoster	Erythroplakia	Drug induced		Xerostomia and
Warts	Neutropenia	Epidermolysis bullosa	Dyskeratosis	Thrombocytopenia		saliva products
Melkersson–	Tuberculosis	Linear IgA disease	congenita			Burning mouth
Rosenthal		Dermatitis	White			syndrome
Sarcoidosis		herpetiformis	sponge naevus			Scleroderma
Heerfordt		Angina bullosa	Submucous			
Angioedema		haemorrhagica	fibrosis			
			Keratosis			
			Hairy leukoplakia			
			Mucositis			
			Candida			

Recommended reading

Bruch JM, Treister NS (2017). *Clinical Oral Medicine and Pathology,* 2nd edition. Cham: Springer.

Greaney L, Brennan PA, Kerawal C, et al. (2014). Why should I follow up my patients with oral lichen planus? *Br J Oral Maxillofac Surg* **52**:291–293.

McCreary CE, McCartan BE (1999). Clinical management of oral lichen planus. *Br J Oral Maxillofac Surg* **37**:338–343.

Scully C (2013). *Oral and Maxillofacial Medicine: The Basis of Diagnosis and Treatment,* 3rd edition. London: Churchill Livingstone.

Scully C, Lo Muzio L (2008). Oral mucosal diseases: mucous membrane pemphigoid. *Br J Oral Maxillofac Surg* **46**:358–366.

Scully C, Mignogna M (2008). Oral mucosal disease: pemphigus. *Br J Oral Maxillofac Surg* **46**:272–277.

Zakrzewska JM (2013a). Multi-dimensionality of chronic pain of the oral cavity and face. *J Headache Pain* **14**:37.

Zakrzewska JM (2013b). Differential diagnosis of facial pain and guidelines for management. *Br J Anaesthesia* **111**(1):95–104.

Zakrzewska JM, Linskey ME (2014). Trigeminal neuralgia. *BMJ* **348**:g474.

Questions in this book

1. Lichen planus.
2. Pemphigus vulgaris.
3. Temporal arteritis.
4. Linear IgA disease.
5. Focal epithelial hyperplasia.
6. Storiform collagenoma.
7. Cat scratch disease.
8. Cluster headaches.
9. Osteoradionecrosis.
10. Medication-related osteonecrosis of the jaws.
11. Intravascular papillary endothelial hyperplasia.
12. Trigeminal neuralgia.
13. Squamous cell carcinoma histology.
14. Malignant transformation.
15. Smoker's melanosis.
16. Drug ulcer.
17. Cavernous sinus thrombosis.
18. Erosive lichen planus.
19. Migraine.
20. Tertiary syphilis.
21. Gingival epulis.
22. Varicella zoster.
23. Premalignant conditions.
24. Dysplasia.
25. Pemphigoid.
26. Burning mouth syndrome.
27. Dyskeratosis congenita.
28. Necrotizing fasciitis.
29. Angular chelitis.
30. Refeeding syndrome.

Craniofacial Surgery

Topics

Assessment	Syndromes	Craniosynostosis	Surgery	Vascular malformations	Others
History Examination Imaging Genetic testing Raised intracranial pressure	Apert Crouzon Gorlin–Goltz Treacher Collins Saethre–Chotzen Pfeiffer	Types, single suture, syndromic Treatment Positional plagiocephaly, torticolis Chiari malformations	Fronto-orbital advancement Le Fort III Monoblock Coronal flap Facial bipartition Box osteotomy Posterior cranial vault remodelling	History Examination Classification Imaging Surgery Embolization Sclerotherapy	Hemifacial microsomia Facial clefting Encephaloceles Cleidocranial dysplasia Craniofacial tumours Thyroglossal duct Craniofacial team Craniofacial services in the UK

Recommended reading

Derderian C, Seaward J (2012). Syndromic craniosynostosis. *Semin Plast Surg* **26**:64–75.

Ehrenfeld M, Neal Futran N, Manson P, Prein J (2020). *Advanced Craniomaxillofacial Surgery. Tumor, Corrective Bone Surgery and Trauma.* Davos: AO Foundation.

Elledge ROC, McMillan K, Monaghan AM, Williams R (2016). Vascular Anomalies. In: Carachi R, Doss S (eds) *Clinical Embryology: An Atlas of Congenital Malformations.* Cham: Springer.

Fowell C, Jones R, Nishikawa H, Monaghan A (2016). Arteriovenous malformations of the head and neck: current concepts in management. *Br J Oral Maxillofac Surg* **54**:482–487.

Fowell C, Verea Linares C, Jones R, et al. (2017). Venous malformations of the head and neck: current concepts in management. *Br J Oral Maxillofac Surg* **55**:3–9.

Hopper RA, Kapadia H, Morton T (2013). Normalising facial ratios in Apert syndrome patients with Le Fort II midface distraction and simultaneous zygomatic repositioning. *Plast Recontr Surg* **132**(1):129–140.

Langdon J, Patel M, Ord R, Brennan P (2017). *Operative Oral and Maxillofacial Surgery*, 3rd edition. Boca Raton: CRC Press.

McCarthy JG, Katzen JT, Hopper R, Grayson BH (2002). The first decade of mandibular distraction: lessons we have learnt. *Plast Recon Surg* **110**(7):1704–1713.

White N, Evans M, Dover MS, et al. (2009). Posterior calvarial vault expansion using distraction osteogenesis. *Childs Nerv Syst* **25**:231–236

Wink JD, Goldstein JA, Paliga JT, et al. (2014). The mandibular deformity in hemifacial microsomia: a reassessment of the Pruzansky and Kaban classification. *Plast Recon Surg* **133**(2):174e–181e.

Questions in this book

1. Treacher Collins syndrome.
2. Vascular tumours.
3. Hemifacial microsomia.

4. Chiari malformation.
5. Lymphatic malformations.
6. Sagittal synostosis.
7. Midface distraction.
8. Gorlin–Goltz.
9. Arteriovenous malformations.
10. Swelling post bleomycin injection.
11. Hemifacial microsomia.
12. The hand in Apert syndrome.
13. Paediatric osteosarcoma.
14. Positional plagiocephaly.
15. Cleidocranial dysplasia.
16. Facial clefting.
17. Treacher Collins.
18. Thyroglossal duct cyst.
19. Posterior cranial vault remodelling.
20. Raised intracranial pressure.

Cleft Surgery

Topics

Assessment	Management	Lip	Palate	Additional surgery	Other
Types	Principles	Straight-line	Von Langenbeck	Nose surgery	Speech and SALT
Aetiology	Timings of	(Rose–Thompson)	Veau	(primary,	Velopharyngeal
Epidemiology	repair	Rotation	Bardach	secondary)	dysfunction
Diagnosis	Surgical	advancement	Furlow	Le Fort	Hearing
Examination	options	(Millard, Delaire)	Sommerlad	I osteotomy	Orthodontics
Investigations	Nose	Z-plasties		(including	Genetic testing
Anatomy of	Fistulae	(Tennison–Randall)		distraction)	Psychology
defects				Bone graft	
				(timing,	
				donor sites)	
				Revision	
				procedures	

Recommended reading

Cheung LK, Chua HDP, Bendeus Hägg M (2006). Cleft maxillary distraction versus orthognathic surgery: clinical morbidities and surgical relapse. *Plast Reconstr Surg* **118**(4):996–1008.

Cutting CB (2000). Secondary cleft lip nasal reconstruction: state of the art. *Cleft Pal Craniofac* **37**(6):538–541.

Demke JC, Tatum SA (2011). Analysis and evolution of rotation principles in unilateral cleft lip repair. *Plast Reconstr Surg* **64**:313–318.

Guyuron B (2008). MOC-PS^{SM} CME article: late cleft lip nasal deformity. *Plast Reconstr Surg* **121**(4):1–11.

Haig R (2009). *Atlas of the Oral and Maxillofacial Surgery Clinics of North America. Cleft Surgery: Repair of the Lip, Palate, and Alveolus*. Philadelphia: Saunders.

Hodgkinson PD, Brown S, Duncan D, et al. (2005). Management of children with cleft lip and palate: a review describing the application of multidisciplinary team working in this condition based upon the experiences of a regional cleft lip and palate centre in the United Kingdom. *Fetal Mat Med Rev* **16**(1):1–27.

Shokrollahi K, Whitaker IS, Laing H (2009). *Multiple Choice Questions in Plastic Surgery*. Shrewsbury: TFM Publishing.

Sommerlad BC (2003). A technique for cleft palate repair. *Plast Reconstr Surg* **112**:1542.

Tibesar RJ, Black A, Sidman JD (2009). Surgical repair of cleft lip and cleft palate. *Op Tech Otolaryngol* **20**:245–255.

Van de Ven B, Defrancq J, Defrancq E (2008). *Cleft Lip Surgery: A Practical Guide*. Marbella: Agave Clinic. https://static1.squarespace.com/static/58d90bbb1e5b6cc3c40786ab/t/58e24e87725e250f9731504f/1491226251547/cleft-lip-book-english.pdf.

Witherow H, Cox S, Jones E, et al. (2002). A new scale to assess radiographic success of secondary alveolar bone grafts. *Cleft Pal Craniofac* **39**(3):255–260.

Questions in this book

1. Goals of cleft surgery.
2. Epidemiology of clefts.
3. Embryology.
4. Speech and resonance.
5. Oronasal fistula.
6. Features of cleft lip.
7. Primary cleft rhinoplasty.
8. Cleft lip repair technique.
9. Alveolar bone grafting.
10. Secondary cleft rhinoplasty.
11. Velopharyngeal dysfunction.
12. Maxillary distraction.
13. Palatal fistula.
14. Cleft maxillary osteotomy.
15. Velopharyngeal dysfunction.

Dentoalveolar Surgery

Topics

Third molars	Canines	Infections	Nerves	Other
Assessment	Assessment	Assessment	Assessment	Flap designs
Imaging including CBCT	Guidelines	Abscess types	Pain classification and syndromes	Autotransplantation
Guidelines	Surgery	Actinomycosis	Repair of damage	Oro-antral fistula (assessment and surgery)
Extraction	Flap design	Fascial space infections	Medicolegal	
Coronectomy	Exposure and bonding	Surgery		
		Ludwig's angina		

Recommended reading

Brennan P, Macleod N (2020). *50 Landmark Papers Every Oral and Maxillofacial Surgeon Should Know.* Boca Raton: CRC Press.

Brennan P, Schliephake H, Ghali GE (2007). *Maxillofacial Surgery,* 3rd edition. London: Churchill Livingstone.

Coulthard P, Bailey E, Esposito M, et al. (2014). Surgical techniques for the removal of mandibular wisdom teeth (review). *Cochrane Dat Sys Rev* **7**:CD004345.

Kushnerev E, Yates JM (2015). Evidence-based outcomes following inferior alveolar and lingual nerve injury and repair: a systematic review *J Oral Rehab* **42**:786–802.

Omran A, Hutchison I, Ridout F, et al. (2020). Current perspectives on the surgical management of mandibular third molars in the United Kingdom: the need for further research. *Br J Oral Maxillofac Surg* 58(3):348–354.

Rapaport BHJ, Brown JS (2020). Systematic review of lingual nerve retraction during surgical mandibular third molar extractions. *Br J Oral Maxillofac Surg* **58**:748–752.

Renton T, Hankins M, Sproate C, McGurk M (2005). A randomised controlled clinical trial to compare the incidence of injury to the inferior alveolar nerve as a result of coronectomy and removal of mandibular third molars. *Br J Oral Maxillofac Surg* **43**:7–12.

Royal College of Surgeons of England (2020). *Clinical Guidelines for Periradicular Surgery.* London: RCS Eng. https://www.rcseng.ac.uk/-/media/files/rcs/fds/publications/periradicular_surgery_guidelines_2020.pdf.

Questions in this book

1. Pericoronitis.
2. Apicectomy.
3. Ludwig's angina.
4. Lingual retraction.
5. Iatrogenic nerve injury.
6. Iatrogenic nerve injury.
7. Iliac crest harvest.
8. Splinting in dental trauma.
9. Oro-antral fistula.
10. Coronectomy.
11. Third molar impaction
12. Dental trauma splint
13. Third molar impaction.
14. Auto transplantation.
15. Ectopic canines.
16. Sensory testing.
17. Risks of third molar surgery.
18. Nerve injury classification.
19. Fibro osseous dysplasia.
20. Facial pain.
21. Oro-antral fistula.
22. Cervicofacial actinomycosis.

23. Bifid mandibular canal.
24. Canine assessment.
25. Tooth necrosis.

Reconstructive Maxillofacial Surgery

Topics

Concepts	Local flaps	Regional flaps	Free flaps	Skin grafts	Bone grafts	Other grafts
Healing	Techniques	Pectoris	Radial	Full thickness	Non-	Nerve
Defect classification	Classification	Deltopectoral	Fibula	Split thickness	vascularized	Cartilage
Quality of life	Principles	Submental	Anterolateral	Dermal matrix	Autogenous	
Reconstructive	Blood supply	island	thigh	substitutes	and alloplastic	
ladder	Nasolabial	Temporalis	DCIA			
	Upper lip		Anastamosis			
	Lower lip		Monitoring			
			Complications			

Recommended reading

Bak M, Jacobson AS, Buchbinder D, Urken ML (2010). Contemporary reconstruction of the mandible. *Oral Oncol* **46**:71–76.

Baker SR (2014). *Local Flaps in Facial Reconstruction*, 3rd edition. Philadelphia: Elsevier.

Balsundaram I, Al-Hadad I, Parmar S (2012). Recent advances in reconstructive oral and maxillofacial surgery. *Br J Oral Maxillofac Surg* **50**:695–705.

Brown J, Bekiroglu F, Shaw R (2010). Indications for the scapular flap in reconstruction of the head and neck. *Br J Oral Maxillofac Surg* **48**:331–337.

Brown JS, Shaw RJ (2010). Reconstruction of the maxilla and midface: introducing a new classification. *Lancet Oncol* **11**:1001–1008.

Chim H, Salgado CJ, Seselgyte R, et al. (2010). Principles of head and neck reconstruction: an algorithm to guide flap selection. *Semin Plast Surg* **24**:148–154.

Fernandez R (2015). *Local and Regional Flaps in Head & Neck Reconstruction. A Practical Approach*. Chichester: Wiley-Blackwell.

Klaus-Dietrich Wolff K, Hölzle F (2018). *Raising of Microvascular Flaps: A Systematic Approach*, 3rd edition. Cham: Springer.

Urken ML, Buchbinder D, Costantino PD, et al. (1998). Oromandibular reconstruction using microvascular composite flaps: report of 210 cases. *Arch Otolaryngol Head Neck Surg* **124**:46–55.

Wei FC, Mardini S (eds) (2009). *Flaps and Reconstructive Surgery*. London: Elsevier.

Questions in this book
1. Temporoparietal flap.
2. Mandible defects.
3. Perforator-based chimeric flap.
4. Mathes and Nahai classification.
5. Partial maxillectomy.

6. Deltopectoral island flap.
7. Fibula flap.
8. Fibula flap.
9. Scapula flap.
10. Fibula flap.
11. Static facial reanimation.
12. Posterior cranial vault remodelling.
13. Paramedian flap.
14. Fibula flap.
15. Free flap monitoring.

Oral Implantology

Topics

Assessment	Planning	Surgical techniques	Materials science	In cancer	Others
History	VSP	Implant drilling	Implant components	In bone flaps	Complications
Risk factors	Single tooth	Flap design	Types	Radiotherapy	Maintenance
Examination	Fixed bridge	Sinus lift	Osseo integration	MRONJ	Microbiology
Imaging	Overdenture	Ridge augmentation		Osteoporosis	Antibiotic prophylaxis
	Aesthetics				
	All-On-4®				

Recommended reading

Chiapasco M, Casentini P, Zaniboni M (2009). Bone augmentation procedures in implant dentistry. *Int J Oral Maxillofac Implants* **24** Suppl:237–259.

Esposito M, Grusovin MG, Felice P, et al. (2009). Interventions for replacing missing teeth: horizontal and vertical bone augmentation techniques for dental implant treatment. *Cochrane Dat Sys Rev* **4**:CD003607.

Ferreira EJ, Kuabara MR, Gulinelli JL (2010). 'All-on-four' concept and immediate loading for simultaneous rehabilitation of the atrophic maxilla and mandible with conventional and zygomatic implants. *Br J Oral Maxillofac Surg* **48**:218–220.

Jensen O (2011). *Oral and Maxillofacial Surgery Clinics of North. Dental Implants*. Volume 23-2. Philadelphia: Saunders.

Malet J (2018). *Implant Dentistry at a Glance*, 2nd edition. Chichester: Wiley-Blackwell.

Questions in this book

1. Bone density.
2. Peri-implantitis.
3. Aesthetics.
4. Implant selection.
5. Microbiology.
6. Antibiotic prophylaxis.
7. The All-On-4® concept.

8. Implant in the maxillary sinus.
9. Implant types.
10. Component loosening.

Aesthetic Facial Surgery

Topics

Assessment	Surgical techniques	Non-surgical techniques	Specific topics
History	Rhinoplasty	Botulinum toxin	Body dysmorphic disorder
Examination	Facelift	Fillers	Implants
Anatomy	Facial reanimation	Chemical peels	Regulation
Signs of aging	Blepharoplasty	Dermabrasion	Training
Investigations	Otoplasty	Microdermabrasion	
	Brow lift	Lasers	
	Liposuction		
	Fat transfer		
	Cheiloplasty		

Recommended reading

Adrian A, Dafydd H (2014). *Key Notes on Plastic Surgery*, 2nd edition. Chichester: Wiley-Blackwell.

Barrett DM, Gerecci D, Wang TD (2016). Facelift controversies. *Facial Plast Surg Clin N Am* **24**:357–366.

Biglioi F (2015a). Facial reanimations: part I—recent paralyses. *Br J Oral Maxillofac Surg* **53**:903–906.

Biglioi F (2015b). Facial reanimations: part II—long-standing paralyses. *Br J Oral Maxillofac Surg* **53**:907–912.

Chiu T (2011). *Stone's Plastic Surgery Facts*, 3rd edition. Cambridge: Cambridge University Press.

Gunter JP, Landecker A, Cochran CS (2006). Frequently used grafts in rhinoplasty: nomenclature and analysis. *Plast Reconstr Surg* **118**(1):14e–29e.

Henk Giele H, Cassell O, Drury P (2016). *Plastic and Reconstructive Surgery. Oxford Specialist Handbooks in Surgery*. Oxford: Oxford University Press.

Hivemaud V, Lefourn B, Robard M, et al. (2017). Autologous fat grafting: a comparative study of four current commercial protocols. *Plast Reconstr Surg* **70**:248–256.

Park SS (2011). Fundamental principles in aesthetic rhinoplasty. *Clin Exp Otorhinolaryngol* **4**(2):55–66.

Richards SD, Jebreel A, Capper R (2009). Otoplasty: a review of the surgical techniques. *Clin Otolaryngol* **30**:2–8.

Shokrollahi M (2009). *Multiple Choice Questions in Plastic Surgery*. Shrewsbury: TFM Publishing.

Weinzweig J (2010). *Plastic Surgery Secrets Plus*, 2nd edition. St Louis: Mosby.

Questions in this book

1. Dorsal hump reduction.
2. Closed tip rhinoplasty.
3. Rhytidectomy.
4. Facelifts.
5. Scar revision.
6. Chemical peels.

7. Facial reanimation.
8. Nasal grafts.
9. Facial reanimation.
10. Ptosis treatment.
11. Burns.
12. Blepharoplasty.
13. Microdermabrasion.
14. Lasers.
15. Otoplasty.

Perioperative Care

Topics

Airway types	Assessment	Clotting	Considerations	Anaesthesia	Medically compromised patients
Cricothyroidotomy Tracheostomy (surgical and percutaneous) Submental intubation Endotracheal intubation	Consent ASA classification Pain WHO checklist Medicolegal	Coagulation Tranexamic acid Blood products Warfarin NOACs	Thromboembolic disease Preventing surgical infections Necrotizing fasciitis Metabolic syndrome Blood test results	General Local Sedation	Steroids Diabetes Infective endocarditis

Recommended reading

Cascarini L, Schilling C, Gurney B, Brennan P (eds) (2018). *Oxford Handbook of Oral and Maxillofacial Surgery,* 2nd edition. Oxford: Oxford University Press.

Questions in this book

1. Hypokalaemia.
2. Cricothyroidotomy.
3. Tranexamic acid
4. Necrotizing fasciitis.
5. Consent.
6. The World Health Organization (WHO) checklist.
7. The American Society of Anesthesiologists (ASA) grading system.
8. Pain medication.
9. Tracheostomy.
10. The airway in patients with Pierre Robin syndrome.

Evidence Based Medicine and Research

Topics

Handling data	Study design	Analysing data	Others
Types	Trials	Single group	Evidence-based medicine
Describing	Cohort	Two related groups	Systematic reviews
Distributions	Case controlled	Two unrelated groups	Cochrane Reviews
Transformations	Randomized	More than two groups	Survival analysis
Sampling		Regression and correlation	Bayesian methods
Statistical measures		Odds ratio	
		Relative risk	

Recommended reading

Greenhalgh T (2019). *How to Read a Paper: The Basics of Evidence-Based Medicine and Healthcare*, 6th edition. Chichester: Wiley-Blackwell.

Petrie A, Sabin C (2019). *Medical Statistics at a Glance*, 4th edition. Chichester: Wiley-Blackwell.

Questions in this book

1. Statistical measures.
2. Types of trials.
3. Odds ratio.
4. Relative risk.
5. Study design.

INTRODUCTION TO THE EXAMINATION

The FRCS (OMFS): the ghost in the machine

When approaching any assessment, it is helpful to put yourself in the mindset of the assessor(s) and understand the parameters (and limitations) of the assessment method being utilized. As a higher surgical trainee, I examined for the Royal College of Physicians and Surgeons of Glasgow and found the insights into the design and delivery of assessments invaluable in conquering my own assessment milestones. Towards the end of my higher training, I worked for a number of years for a private company that specialized in 'coaching' doctors to succeed at job interviews. The innate understanding of the methods behind shaping the ideal interview and scoring prospective employees enabled me to effectively 'second guess' any interviewer. Understanding the process (and challenges) behind setting a written assessment will hopefully equip you with similar insights and enable you to optimize your preparation.

Utility

In my capacity as a module lead for an undergraduate degree, if the results are returned and everyone has passed the end-of-year examination, there is a tendency to breathe a sigh of relief. There will be no emails of complaint or appeal, no need to produce a supplementary examination, and students will progress uneventfully to the next academic year with the minimum degree of fuss. And then some nagging doubts creep in. Was the assessment fit for purpose? Was it discerning of who 'deserved' to achieve a pass? Are we sure that everyone has 'measured up' to a level that can be regarded as safe and competent in the real world? In short, was it too easy?

Candidates for the Fellowship of the Royal College of Surgeons in Oral & Maxillofacial Surgery FRCS (OMFS) who fail the assessment may find themselves lamenting two things: that the exam was 'too difficult' and that it was 'unfair'. But these are two very different concepts. The former may be true, but if everyone is of a similar standard, then all candidates should find the assessment equally 'difficult'. This is the purpose of **standard setting**. The term 'unfair' should hopefully never be applied to such a high-stakes assessment, as the exam should be appropriately **blueprinted** against a syllabus and also exhibit a number of key characteristics:

- **reliability** (that we can 'trust' the results);
- **validity** (that the assessment assesses what it purports to assess);
- **acceptability** (that all stakeholders are comfortable with the method chosen);
- **educational impact** (that the assessment is of inherent value in driving development of candidates);

- **cost effectiveness**; and
- **practicability** (that the resources exist to deliver the assessment).

All of these factors translate into an overarching concept of **utility** (van der Vleuten 1996).

You can already see how attractive a written assessment such as the first part of the FRCS (OMFS) is in terms of some of these features. It costs little and it is appreciably practicable to herd candidates into a local driving test centre and seat them in front of computers. They are likely to accept it without complaint, having had years of sitting similar written assessments such that the format is a familiar one. The promise (or possibly the threat!) of covering the breadth of the syllabus will prompt candidates to revise it in its entirety, arguably driving them to ensure that they have the requisite knowledge. But how valid and reliable is it?

SBA writing (and reverse engineering for success)

The FRCS examination now exclusively uses the single best answer (SBA) format of questioning, reflecting a wider move in this regard across undergraduate and postgraduate medical education. Systems such as **Bloom's taxonomy** (Bloom et al. 1956) and **Miller's pyramid** (Miller 1990) describe different levels of cognition that can be assessed, ranging from simple factual recall to exercising judgement in applying knowledge to real clinical dilemmas. It is tempting to see SBAs as simply a means of testing knowledge recall, but this would arguably constitute a poor use of a question type that has superseded other multiple choice question (MCQ) formats such as Extended Matching Items (EMIs), Key-Features Items (KFIs), and Script Concordance Items (SCIs).

Well-written SBAs should test higher-order thinking in differentiating between the correct response and a number of plausible distractors that are *less* correct (but not necessarily incorrect). At such a stage in training, one may argue that no single person is the arbiter of the *most* correct answer in some clinical dilemmas (or that there is a single correct response for some problems). The key here is second-guessing the intention from the question, with the information provided in the **stem** (the opening paragraph that 'sets the scene') of an SBA. The rest of the ambiguity should be 'weeded out' by standard setting and **post-exam analysis**.

The strategy for writing a good SBA should include a stem that demonstrates the following qualities:

- It should address a single problem.
- It should be worded positively.
- It should contain only relevant information.
- The question can be answered without reference to the alternative options by a proficient candidate.

The options then provided (the correct answer with four possible distractors) should demonstrate the following attributes:

- They should be homogenous.
- They should be mutually exclusive.
- All possible answers should be plausible.
- The range of options should prevent candidates who *don't* know the answer from guessing correctly.
- They should also prevent candidates who *do* know the answer from being confused.
- There should be balanced placement of the correct answer throughout the exam paper.
- Possible answers should ideally exclude similar terms to the stem (avoidance of clues).

Good questions overall avoid absolutes (e.g. 'always' or 'never'); they have stems; their options are grammatically and syntactically consistent; and they avoid options such as 'all of the above' (the candidate only needs to recognize two correct answers) and 'none of the above' (the assessor will never know if the candidate knew the correct answer!).

Examiners, like all of us, are fallible. The system is robust, but one can see how there might be a number of potential 'loopholes' when faced with the question that one genuinely cannot fathom. Whilst the authors of this work hope that you will use it to become the very best clinician your patients deserve, for that small minority of questions that are a source of genuine quandary, the following 'tricks' can be reverse engineered from failure in ideal question writing:

- Convergence strategy (within an exam paper, questions covering similar ground may 'hint' at the answers of each other).
- Choose one of two polar opposites among the options (second-guessing the question writer's desire to hide the correct answer).
- Ignore offers of 'x only' and 'y only' if 'x+y' is available.
- Choose the most elaborate answer (this being the one the question writer put most thought into).
- Choose 'none of the above' or 'all of the above' if on offer.
- Select the answer cued by the stem (e.g. the only 'treatment' among 'management options' when the question asks for a 'treatment').
- Avoid options containing absolutes (e.g. 'always' or 'never').
- Choose the answer written in the idiosyncratic style of a known examiner with a 'hobby horse', e.g. particular phraseology.

When all else fails, choose the middle option! In all seriousness, these strategies are last resorts and a robust and well-written examination will have undermined these strategies! But they are worth bearing in mind when faced with the question that seems impossible to answer.

Standard setting

In terms of reliability, an SBA paper allows a degree of **temporal stability** (comparable performance on different occasions—although many candidates will say some sittings were more difficult than others) and assessment of **internal consistency** (that all the questions contribute to a meaningful global assessment of a candidate). There should be a degree of professional embarrassment among examiners rather than pride in writing the question that examines inconsequential minutiae of knowledge that bears no relevance to clinical practice. Arguably such a question has no place in the exam and should be screened out at the standard setting hurdle or in a post-exam analysis.

There are various methods of standard setting an examination. Standards may be **absolute or criterion-referenced**, whereby there is a set level of competence to be achieved, below which a candidate fails. The alternative is **relative or norm-referenced** standards, whereby the level is set by the performance of the group. Arguably, a combination would be best, ensuring that the possibility exists for all candidates to reach a standard, which might be flexible given the inherent temporal instability. In my undergraduate module I use the **Cohen method**. This is based on the premise of defining the 'cut score' as 60% of the grade achieved by the 95th percentile candidate. It is inexpensive, easy to apply, and a reasonable representation of group performance, whilst excluding outliers (the 'genius' beyond the 95th percentile). For a high-stakes examination such as the FRCS (OMFS), however, this will not do.

The FRCS (OMFS) uses the **modified Angoff method** (Angoff 1971). For such a small number of candidates sitting such a career-defining assessment, this is ideal. Effectively, examiners review each SBA to determine what would be the probability of a borderline candidate answering the question correctly, expressed from 0 to 1 (where 1 equates to all 'just passing' candidates choosing the correct response). The individual SBA probabilities are added up for each examiner and all of these scores are then summed together to arrive at a total. This, divided by the number of examiners, determines the percentage 'cut score' for the exam.

The method produces reliable judgements determined by content differences and enables past assessment results to inform examiner judgements on performances (Norcini and McKinley 2005). This latter point is key when only a handful of candidates are sitting the exam each year. The problem can be perceived, however, that having a minimum level of years as a specialist to become an examiner translates to a panel of experts who cannot quite recall their first day as a consultant! As such, the temptation for scoffing and muttering that everyone should know the answer to the esoteric SBA question before them quickly translates into an inordinately high pass mark. Just as with question design, standard setting works when applied *properly*. The good news is you are all in it together with the other candidates, both now and in the past, in determining the threshold for a pass.

Post-exam analysis and quality assurance

When the dust has settled, and everyone has shuffled exhausted from the driving centre to the pub or coffee shop down the road, negativity bias will prompt a recall of *that* question. It's the one no one could answer, or that everyone had a different answer for. And you would be forgiven for thinking that you have to count that as a mark lost. But, maybe not.

The statistics after the event enable the final decision-making about questions that should be excluded from this examination and potentially all future sittings. **Point biserial coefficients** enable examiners to see how well individual questions correlated with performance on the assessment overall. Methods of analysis such as **twenty percentile histograms** for individual questions, **33% item discrimination**, and the **Kuder–Richardson formula** all serve to augment this and inform an impression of reliability. Value also comes from 'eyeballing' the item analysis for each question. If a disproportionate number of candidates return the incorrect answer, or a question proves divisive in terms of the weighting of responses received, then arguably such a question should be closely examined to ascertain whether it is fit for purpose or a product of a biased (and potentially incorrect) opinion of the author. Great trainers learn plenty from their trainees, who are fantastic cross-pollinators of ideas and concepts, and the quality assurance process of post-exam question analysis is no exception. Next time candidates are undermining each other's confidence in the post-exam wind down, they would do well to remember this!

The way forward

Surgical training has moved with the times and continues to develop in terms of delivery and assessment of the art and science. Performance-based tasks, self-assessment, portfolios, and a focus on 'softer skills' in the apprenticeship that is higher surgical training all evidence progressive thinking, with an evidence base in training the surgeons of tomorrow. In time, hopefully, we will move even further in asking not just what surgeons can do, but who they are fundamentally as individuals with a well-calibrated moral compass (Elledge et al. 2020).

Amongst all these changes, written examinations such as the initial part of the FRCS can be seen as somewhat archaic, but they still have their place. They have a number of advantages, as can be seen, but arguably there is a technique to passing them beyond simple knowledge retention, which seems to play into the hands of some candidates' abilities to 'second guess' examiners' intentions better than their peers. Hopefully this chapter will have afforded you some insights into the method behind the madness, and the remainder of this book will enable you rehearse the technique of answering well-constructed SBA questions reflective of the exam itself. Remember, it is real clinical judgement we (and hopefully the examiners) are after, and with just over 60 precious seconds per question, there is room for little else. Above and beyond the tips and tricks, remember the principle of Occam's razor, that sometimes the simplest explanation is the best. Examiners (with a few exceptions!) assume the role to make sure the people are ready to start a long and fruitful career in the specialty. As such, more often than not, they are asking reasonable questions in a reasonable way and not trying to catch you out!

References

Angoff WH (1971). Scales, norms and equivalent scores. In: Thorndike RL, Angoff WH, Lindquist EF, American Council on Education (eds) *Educational Measurement*, 2nd edition, 508–600. Washington, DC: American Council on Education.

Bloom BS, Englehart MD, Furst EJ, Hill WH, Krathwohl DR (1956). *A Taxonomy of Educational Objectives: Handbook I: Cognitive Domain*. New York: David McKay.

Elledge R, Brennan P, Mohamud A, Jones J (2020). Phronesis and virtue ethics: the future of surgical training? *British Journal of Oral and Maxillofacial Surgery* **58**(2):125–128.

Miller G (1990). The assessment of clinical skills/competence/performance. *Academic Medicine* **65**(Suppl):S63–S67.

Norcini J, McKinley DW (2005). Concepts in assessment including standard setting. In: Harden RM, Dent JA (eds) *A Practical Guide for Medical Teachers*, 252–259. London: Churchill Livingstone.

van der Vleuten CPM (1996). The assessment of professional competence: developments, research and practical implications. *Advances in Health Sciences Education* **1**: 41–67.

1. **All the following types of external radiation therapy help to reduce radiation damage to normal tissues with the exception of which *one* of the following?**
   A. Three-dimensional conformal radiation therapy
   B. Image-guided radiation therapy
   C. Helical-tomotherapy
   D. Intensity-modulated radiation therapy (IMRT)
   E. Photon beam radiation therapy

2. **The day after a bilateral type one modified radical neck dissection, a patient is noticed to have a diastolic blood pressure of 100 mmHg and increased facial swelling. Which of the following is false?**
   A. Immediate management includes elevation of the head.
   B. The patient will likely have facial swelling
   C. The patient should be investigated pre-operatively with digital subtraction angiography
   D. This clinical picture may be associated with increased intracranial pressure (ICP)
   E. This complication would be prevented by staged neck dissections

3. **You are asked to provide an opinion of a patient struggling to eat following treatment for primary tonsil carcinoma. They are losing weight but are currently able to tolerate oral feed. Which of the following statements is true?**
   A. The patient likely has stage 3 mucositis
   B. The patient should be started on nasogastric feeding
   C. The mucositis is due to radiotherapy (RT)
   D. The mainstay of treatment is with alcohol-based barrier products
   E. Oral rinses are encouraged over toothbrushing to decrease irritation

4. **A 45-year-old patient is referred from her dentist with an inflammatory mass extruding from a recently extracted upper molar tooth socket. She has altered sensation to her cheek. Computed tomography (CT) scan demonstrates a mass that extends into the ipsilateral ethmoid sinus but no regional or distant spread. Which of the following statements is true?**
    A. This patient has stage 4 disease
    B. Extension onto the pterygoid plates is likely
       C. Disease has a worse prognosis than similar disease originating in the adjacent palatal mucosa
    D. Adjuvant RT is only required if pathology demonstrates adenoid cystic carcinoma
    E. Elective neck dissection of levels 1–4 should be performed due to a high risk of local metastasis

5. **Within the *AJCC Cancer Staging Manual, Eighth Edition*, which of the following classifications for oral cancer is true?**
    A. pTNM refers to the post-treatment classification
    B. ypTNM is the post-therapy pathological classification
    C. pTNM is utilized when chemoradiotherapy is the primary treatment modality
    D. rTNM is used for all patients with cancer identified before treatment
    E. aTNM is the alternative classification for previously undiagnosed oral cancers

6. **A 73-year-old patient presents with a 3-cm-wide squamous cell carcinoma (SCC) of the upper lip extending into the commissure. Incisional biopsy demonstrated invasion of 4 mm and the presence of minor salivary glands. Which of the following is false?**
    A. The Abbe-Estlander flap is commonly used in reconstruction
    B. Staging with CT is not required
    C. Two-year survival would be expected to be approximately 70%
    D. Primary radiochemotherapy is more commonly used than had it presented on the tongue
    E. Brachytherapy is an accepted treatment modality

7. **You review the recipient site of a recent split skin graft. The graft has fully taken but appears dry. Which of the following about the way in which this graft heals is true?**
    A. It may grow hair if complete take occurs
    B. Plasmatic imbibition starts at day three
    C. Inosculation starts at day two
    D. Re-innervation may result in sweating
    E. Success is primarily dependent upon graft thickness

8. **You are awaiting the start of an elective lymph node biopsy for an otherwise healthy patient who is suspected of having lymphoma. The anaesthetic team have failed oral intubation. They have placed a supraglottic airway but ventilation is suboptimal. They have resorted to bag valve mask ventilation. Which is the most appropriate decision at this stage?**
   A. Wake the patient up
   B. Intubate the trachea via the supraglottic airway
   C. Needle cricothyroidotomy
   D. Surgical cricothyroidotomy
   E. Surgical tracheostomy

9. **Which of the following statements regarding IMRT is true?**
   A. It is now used for all patients undergoing RT for head and neck squamous cell carcinoma (HNSCC)
   B. The total dose is commonly 60 Gray (Gy)
   C. Volumetric-modulated arc RT varies in that the machine rotates around the patient during an RT beam in an arc shape
   D. It utilizes two-dimensional conformational RT techniques
   E. It enables identical doses of radiation to be given across the tumour

10. **Which of the following is true regarding chemotherapy for the treatment of oral cancer?**
    A. Chemotherapy has a direct tumoricidal effect at the local primary site in the oral cavity
    B. Chemotherapy is now given routinely for all T2 oral cancers without nodal involvement due to the survival benefit it confers
    C. Its radiosensitizing effect reduces mitotic activity in cancer cells
    D. Induction chemotherapy negates the need for subsequent chemotherapy with RT
    E. The response seen to neoadjuvant chemotherapy is independent to the response to later treatment

11. **Which of the following is true regarding chemoradiotherapy in the treatment of locally advanced head and neck cancer?**
    A. It confers a survival benefit of approximately 6.5% at 5 years independent of RT
    B. Chemotherapy alone should be given for distant metastases, but does not significantly extend survival
    C. Cetuximab provides less toxicity than standard chemotherapy agents such as cisplatin
    D. There is a survival benefit of giving neoadjuvant rather than concurrent chemotherapy with RT
    E. Human papillomavirus (HPV) positive status alters chemotherapy management regimens

12. **Following fine needle aspiration cytology (FNAC) of a thyroid lesion, which one of the following is the recommended correct decision?**
    A. For a Thy 1 result, FNAC should be repeated with ultrasound guidance
    B. For a Thy 2 result, a biopsy should be repeated in 12 months
    C. Complete thyroidectomy is required for all Thy 3 lesions
    D. Surgery is indicated for a Thy4 lesion, as it is diagnostic of malignancy
    E. Thy 5 cytology reflects a 99% positive predictive value for malignancy on subsequent histology

13. **Prior to performing an orbital floor repair on a 35-year-old man injured in a road traffic collision, the anaesthetist incidentally notes a neck lump just to the side of the midline. A review of the original CT scan taken in the emergency department following the initial injury demonstrates thyroid nodules. An ultrasound performed 2 weeks later is reported as a U2 thyroid lesion. Which of the following is false?**
    A. Fine needle aspiration (FNA) is required
    B. The nodules on the CT scan necessitate treatment
    C. Indeterminate lesions should have repeat ultrasound only
    D. A U4 lesion is malignant
    E. A U5 lesion necessitates magnetic resonance imaging (MRI)

14. **Last week you undertook an incisional biopsy of a suspicious lesion affecting the lateral tongue. The biopsy report demonstrates a 3.5-cm area of non-keratinizing SCC incorporating tonsil tissue. CT scan demonstrates no cervical lymphadenopathy. Which of the following is false?**
    A. Primary treatment with radical RT of levels II–IV is recommended
    B. A histopathologic clearance of at least 5 mm is recommended
    C. This type of SCC is uncommon in this location
    D. Transoral surgery and neck dissection is recommended
    E. The pathological features of this SCC suggest improved survival rates compared to other types of SCC

15. **A 60-year-old patient with known ischaemic heart disease (IHD) is awaiting surgery for a stage 3 SCC of the tongue. He takes clopidogrel, enalapril, and atorvastatin. He recently finds that he is increasingly tired and breathless after walking up one flight of stairs. Which of the following is true?**
    A. He requires urgent cardiology referral
    B. Clopidogrel should be discontinued 5 days pre-operatively
    C. National guidelines advise there is no need to stop Dabigatran pre-operatively
    D. The tiredness is a likely side effect of the statin
    E. Enalapril should be given on the day of surgery

16. In which of these cases would a CT scan be least likely to be required to supplement an MRI for the assessment of the primary tumour site?

A. An oral cavity lesion in the retromolar trigone

B. A 1-cm lesion of the posterior tongue visible on nasendoscopy

C. A large mucoepidermoid parotid gland lesion

D. A hypopharyngeal lesion presenting with dysphagia

E. A lesion occluding a posterior sphenoid sinus

17. A 60-year-old woman presents with a 2-month history of a firm painless submandibular swelling. The skin overlying the swelling feels attached to the mandible beneath. Intraoral and extraoral examination demonstrates no pathology. What investigation would you do next?

A. MR scan

B. Positron emission tomography (PET) scan

C. CT scan

D. Excisional lymph node biopsy

E. Bilateral diagnostic tonsillectomy

18. A 65-year-old woman with recently treated cancer is referred by her oncologist with altered sensation in her right lower lip and alteration in the fit of her partial denture. Which of the following is the single best answer?

A. A radiograph will most likely demonstrate a punched-out radiolucency in the posterior mandible

B. Oral examination will likely demonstrate a submucosal mass in the anterior mandible

C. This is most commonly seen in stage 1 breast cancer

D. The lesion occurs due to the large proportion of red marrow

E. The lesion most likely originates from the liver

19. For which of the treatment choices should Quality of Life (QoL) decisions be considered when treating biopsy-proven SCC of the head and neck?

A. Radical RT versus transoral surgery for an early stage tonsil lesion

B. Concurrent chemotherapy in a 65-year-old patient

C. Laser excision rather than primary RT for an early stage laryngeal lesion

D. RT versus excision for stage 2 mucocutaneous lesion of the lip

E. Elective neck dissection for an HPV positive lateral tongue lesion in a 30-year-old patient

20. **With regard to TNM staging, which of the following about nodal involvement by SCC is true?**
    A. Isolated tumour cells (ITCs) are collections of cells less than 1 mm in diameter
    B. A micrometastasis is defined as a tumour deposit between 0.2 and 2 mm in diameter
    C. A conventional metastasis is a tumour deposit more than 1 cm in diameter
    D. The number of positive nodes provides greater prognostic information than extracapsular spread
    E. The presence of ITCs signifies stage 3 disease

21. **A 40-year-old patient with persistent dysphonia undergoes flexible nasendoscopy in clinic which demonstrates a right vocal cord lesion but normal cord mobility. Biopsy demonstrates SCC. MRI head and neck shows a unilateral tumour extending into the supraglottis, but no enlarged neck nodes. Which of the following is true?**
    A. This is staged as T2bN0M0
    B. Right-sided elective neck dissection (END) or RT to levels III–VI is recommended
    C. Transoral laser microsurgery is recommended over RT
    D. Endoscopic examination of the larynx, pharynx, and upper oesophagus should be undertaken at the time of biopsy
    E. RT should be avoided with the exception of treating recurrence, as this commonly causes permanent dysphonia and odynophagia

22. **Which of the following is false about the role of sentinel lymph node biopsy (SLNB) in biopsy-proven oral SCC?**
    A. SLNB is recommended if staged T3N0
    B. SLNB should be offered for a T2 lateral tongue being treated by laser excision without reconstruction
    C. Use of SLNB is institution dependent in the UK
    D. SLNB has a negative predictive value of over 90%
    E. SLNB provides greater information on micrometastasis and extracapsular spread than standard END

23. **Which of the following is not an indication for adjuvant RT following neck dissection in oral SCC?**
    A. T3 or T4 primary lesion
    B. Extracapsular extension
    C. N1 neck disease
    D. Histological pattern of invasion
    E. Perineural invasion

24. **A 77-year-old patient presents with the image shown in Figure 2.1. On imaging, the lesion is 3 cm in diameter and there is a 2-cm ipsilateral neck node in level II. The patient undergoes hemiglossectomy plus unilateral selective neck dissection (SND) of levels I–IV. Which of the following is the *least* appropriate treatment next?**

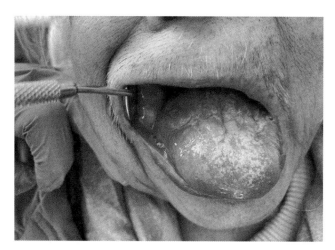

Figure 2.1 Appearance of the tongue on first presentation prior to surgery.

    A. If positive margins are found in the tongue excision, the patient should have chemotherapy or RT

    B. If multiple positive nodes are found after SND then subsequent RT is appropriate

    C. If no adverse features are found after SND then no further treatment is required

    D. If a positive node is found after SND in level IV then chemoradiation is appropriate

    E. If extra-capsular spread (ECS) is demonstrated on SND then she should have chemoradiotherapy

25. **Which of the following statements is correct regarding lymph node level boundaries, content, and drainage?**

    A. Nodes lying medial to the carotid arteries above the level of the hyoid bone are part of level II

    B. The posterior part of the submandibular triangle contains the external carotid artery

    C. Level III nodes radiologically are those anterior to the anterior edge of the SCM and lateral to the lateral margin of the common carotid arteries

    D. Level IV nodes most often contain metastatic deposits from malignancies of the hypopharynx, thyroid, and oral cavity

    E. Level V is divided into a and b by the inferior edge of the hyoid bone

26. **A 38-year-old patient presents with an isolated enlarged level 2 neck node. CT and MRI show no other lesions. Ultrasound-guided fine needle biopsy demonstrates SCC. PET–CT is negative. Which is *not* an appropriate next step?**
   A. Guided biopsy
   B. Narrow-band imaging endoscopy
   C. Tongue base mucosectomy
   D. Nodal pathology should be confirmed by open surgical biopsy
   E. Bilateral tonsillectomy

27. **A 69-year-old man presents with a large unilateral neck swelling as shown in Figure 2.2. He had a T4N1M0 tongue base SCC previously treated with RT. CT scan now demonstrates multiple enlarged unilateral neck nodes with circumferential involvement of the common carotid. Pus is draining from a cutaneous sinus. He has severe IHD, and diabetes necessitating insulin, and his wife informs you that over the last few months he can no longer climb the stairs and is sleeping on the sofa in their front room. Which of the following is true?**

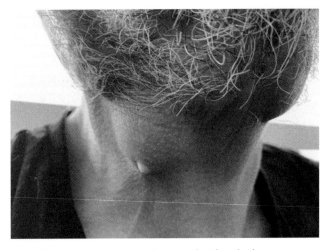

Figure 2.2 Neck swelling in a patient previously treated with radiotherapy.

   A. Treatment should include cisplatin, cetuximab, and 5-fluorouracil (5-FU)
   B. Patients presenting such as this are not suitable for clinical trials of novel chemotherapeutic agents
   C. A type 1 modified radical neck dissection is recommended to treat the neck disease
   D. Salvage surgical treatment should be offered
   E. His performance status is more important than his comorbidities in terms of prognostication

28. **You review a patient with T4N2M1 oral cancer who has bulky inoperable neck disease with circumferential tracheal involvement. She is finding it progressively more difficult to breath and is in pain from her spinal metastases. Which is the *least* appropriate for symptom control?**
    A. Surgical tracheostomy
    B. RT to the spine
    C. Debulking surgery
    D. 5-FU and cisplatin
    E. Bisphosphonates

29. **In which scenario is the procedure shown in Figure 2.3 superior to FNA in the diagnosis of malignancies within the thyroid gland?**

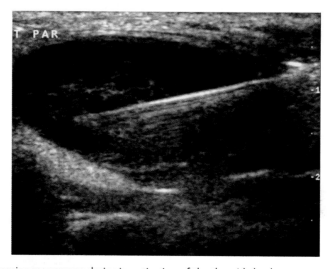

Figure 2.3 Imaging appearance during investigation of the thyroid gland.

    A. Anaplastic thyroid carcinoma from thyroid lymphoma
    B. Papillary thyroid cancer from anaplastic thyroid carcinoma
    C. Follicular thyroid carcinoma from papillary thyroid carcinoma
    D. Medullary thyroid carcinoma from anaplastic thyroid carcinoma
    E. Follicular thyroid carcinoma from medullary thyroid carcinoma

30. **During surgical resection of head and neck cancer, sacrifice of which of the following cranial nerves is unlikely to affect swallowing?**
    A. 5
    B. 7
    C. 10
    D. 11
    E. 12

1. **E. Photon beam radiation therapy.** Photon beam radiation therapy is another name for what is usually known as external beam radiation therapy. Photons are fired by a linear accelerator to get to the tumour but also can damage healthy tissue around it. Proton beams on the other hand may be able to deliver more radiation to the tumour while reducing side effects on normal tissues.

2. **E. This would be prevented by staged neck dissections.** This patient has had bilateral neck dissections that only preserve the spinal accessory nerves. Bilateral internal jugular vein resection can lead to venous congestion and facial swelling. Raised ICP occurs with secondary systemic hypertension (Cushing's reflex). This rise in ICP commonly requires aggressive treatment with hyperventilation, fluid restriction, steroids, and mannitol. The ICP frequently returns to normal within 24 hours. There can be a significant rise in ICP in a staged second neck dissection even if the subsequent operation is undertaken many years after the initial surgery.

3. **A. The patient likely has stage 3 mucositis.** The World Health Organization Oral Toxicity score classifies oral mucositis into 0–4. Patients who can still tolerate a liquid oral diet are classed as stage 3 and should be kept on this medium. Although RT is the most common cause in a patient with treated oropharyngeal cancer (50% of patients), it can occur with chemotherapy agents such as 5-FU (10–15%).

4. **C. Disease has a worse prognosis than similar disease originating in the adjacent palatal mucosa.** This patient has stage 2 invasive SCC originating from the maxillary sinus. Treatment is by maxillectomy, but END is not routinely performed. For stage II cancers and stage I cancers that couldn't be removed completely, had positive margins, or had perineural invasion, post-operative adjuvant radiation is generally given.

5. **B. aTNM is the alternative classification for previously undiagnosed oral cancers.** The classification ypTNM is used when the first therapy is systemic and/or radiation therapy and is followed by surgery. pTNM is the pathological classification used for patients if surgery is the first definitive therapy. rTNM is recurrence or retreatment classification used for assigning stage at time of recurrence or progression until treatment is initiated. aTNM is used for cancers not previously recognized that are found as an incidental finding at autopsy.

6. **D. Primary radiochemotherapy is more commonly used than had it presented on the tongue.** This is false. This patient presents with stage 2 oral SCC of the lip. Primary radiochemotherapy is less commonly utilized than other head and neck sites. Brachytherapy as sole treatment can produce cure rates equivalent to surgery. Imaging of early stage tumours of the lip is usually not indicated.

7. **C. Inosculation starts at day two.** A split thickness skin graft comprises all of the epidermis and dermis and therefore contains sweat glands, sebaceous glands, and hair follicles.

A split skin graft will therefore be dry and lack hair. Plasmatic imbibition precedes inosculation, with graft take primarily dependent upon the extent and speed at which vascular perfusion is restored.

8. D. Surgical cricothyroidotomy. This is an unanticipated difficult airway scenario, in a patient that does not need life or death surgery. However, as the patient cannot be intubated or ventilated, according to the UK Difficult Airway Society guidelines published in 2015, you should proceed to surgical cricothyroidotomy.

9. C. Volumetric-modulated arc RT varies in that the machine rotates around the patient during an RT beam in an arc shape. IMRT is the accepted standard RT for patients undergoing primary and adjuvant RT for head and neck squamous cell carcinoma (HNSCC) except T1/T2N0 glottic cancer. It enables different doses of radiation to be given across the tumour. The international standard for definitive treatment remains 70 Gy, although many centres in the UK use 65 Gy in daily fractions of 2 Gy over 7 weeks. Three-dimensional conformational RT techniques are standard for RT to the head and neck cancer region.

10. A. Chemotherapy has a direct tumoricidal effect at the local primary site in the oral cavity. Chemotherapy is not given routinely for early primary T1/T2 disease without nodal involvement. If given with RT it can have a radiosensitizing effect, making cancer cells more susceptible to RT and increasing the cancer cell kill. If induction chemotherapy is used, further chemotherapy is usually given with subsequent RT, and this is known as sequential chemotherapy. The response to neoadjuvant chemotherapy could give important prognostic information, as it can act as a surrogate marker for response to later treatment.

11. B. Chemotherapy alone should be given for distant metastases, but does not significantly extend survival. In the Meta-analysis of Chemotherapy in Head and Neck Cancer (MACH-NC) trial the use of chemotherapy plus RT provided an additional survival benefit when added to RT alone (6.5% decrease in mortality at 5 years). Cisplatin gives different toxic side effects than standard chemotherapy agents, but, overall, they are of similar severity. The potential benefit of neoadjuvant or induction chemotherapy is being re-examined now, but most recent work has not shown a substantial benefit. At present, HPV status does not alter management regimens, although there are multiple studies underway examining if less intense treatment, both with RT and chemotherapy, could be given to achieve the same outcome but with less toxicity.

12. E. Thy 5 cytology reflects a 99% positive predictive value for malignancy on subsequent histology. For a non-diagnostic result (Thy 1), an ultrasound should be requested with or without repeat FNAC. For a Thy 2 result, two diagnostic benign results 3–6 months apart are required to exclude neoplasia. A Thy 4 result is abnormal and suspicious (but not diagnostic) of papillary, medullary, or anaplastic carcinoma.

13. A. FNA is required. According to the 2014 revised British Thyroid Association guidelines for the management of thyroid cancer, for U1–2 lesions on ultrasound, FNA is not required unless the lesion is high risk. High-risk factors include being a male under age 40 or a history of radiation therapy to the head or neck. U3–5 lesions should have US-guided FNA. Incidental nodules on CT scan only require FNA in high-risk groups.

14. C. This type of SCC is uncommon in this location. This statement is false. The lingual tonsils are located on the posterior aspect of the tongue and therefore this patient is treated as an oropharyngeal cancer. Typical HPV-associated carcinomas are non-keratinizing (basaloid) carcinomas. The status of HPV is a strong and independent prognostic factor for survival, but does not affect which treatment modality should be chosen, although clinical trials are currently underway. Transoral surgery and END or alternatively radical RT to levels II–IV is recommended for T2N0 oropharyngeal SCC. Resection with a clinical margin of 10 mm is recommended to aim for histopathologic clearance of at least 5 mm.

15. A. He requires urgent cardiology referral. According to the document 'Pre-treatment clinical assessment in head and neck cancer', patients with poorly controlled or unstable IHD should be referred for cardiology assessment pre-operatively. Clopidogrel should be discontinued 7 days pre-operatively but Warfarin 5 days before. Newer oral anticoagulants (e.g. Dabigatran and Apixaban) have variable elimination times depending on renal and liver function, but no national guidelines exist for how they should be managed pre-operatively. Angiotensin-converting enzyme inhibitors should be withheld on the day of surgery unless they are for the treatment of heart failure.

16. B. A 1-cm lesion of the posterior tongue visible on nasendoscopy. The preferred imaging modality for all primary malignancies in the head and neck is MRI. Small or subclinical primaries in the tonsil and tongue base that present with cervical lymphadenopathy can be difficult to identify with all forms of imaging including PET–CT. For oral cavity lesions adjacent to the alveolus, MRI should be supplemented by CT to aid assessment of cortical invasion. In those patients who have difficulty with swallowing, aspiration, or breathing when supine, a CT scan will need to be strongly considered. Perineural or skull base involvement most commonly occurs in adenoid cystic and mucoepidermoid carcinoma and often requires a combined multimodality CT and MR approach.

17. A. MR scan. This patient has cervical lymph node with no obvious origin and you should start down the unknown primary pathway by requesting an MR scan. MR is slightly better than CT in such cases as it may identify small high signal intensity lesions in the tonsils and posterior tongue that may metastasize to the submandibular area. A PET scan is subsequently undertaken if no obvious pathology is identified on an MR scan. US-guided core biopsy of the node should be performed instead of excision; this core biopsy is better than FNA as it may provide the HPV and Epstein–Barr virus (EBV) status, which in turn may point to a potential primary lesion.

18. B. Oral examination will likely demonstrate a submucosal mass in the anterior mandible. This patient most likely has metastases to the mandible. These are most commonly present as submucosal lumps, arising from the breast, prostate, lungs, and kidneys. Presence of teeth seems to be an important determinant on oral site preference for metastases. The mandible has little active marrow, especially as we age. Although the most common radiological appearance is a discrete radiolucency, it is not classically punched out.

19. E. Elective neck dissection for an HPV positive lateral tongue lesion in a 30-year-old patient. According to the QoL considerations in head and neck cancer guidelines, QoL is becoming increasingly important for making decisions for the optimal treatment of head and neck cancer in which two treatment modalities have equal outcomes, including survival. Although outcomes for HPV positive lesions are better, currently there is insufficient evidence to support de-escalation of treatment. Although older patients do have a slightly increased survival advantage with concurrent chemotherapy, its use must be carefully considered as it comes with significant QoL issues. Early stage lip cancer can be treated equally well by surgery or radiation therapy.

20. B. A micrometastasis is defined as a tumour deposit between 0.2 and 2 mm in diameter. According to the pathological aspects of the assessment of head and neck cancers guidelines, the terminology of possible nodal involvement by carcinoma is carefully detailed to avoid confusion. ITCs are collections of cells less than 0.2 mm in diameter. A conventional metastasis is a tumour deposit greater than 2 mm in diameter. Extracapsular spread provides greater prognostic information than the number of positive nodes. In terms of TNM staging, the presence of ITCs is currently classified as pN0, as their significance is unknown.

21.   D. Endoscopic examination of the larynx, pharynx, and upper oesophagus should be undertaken at the time of biopsy.   The stage of this disease is currently T2aN0, and a CT scan of the thorax and abdomen is required to assess distant disease. For T2a disease, in the absence of nodal disease, elective treatment of the neck (RT or surgery +/− post-operative RT) is not recommended. A Cochrane Review by Dey et al. (2002) demonstrated that both RT and transoral laser microsurgery have equal survival rates in the treatment of early glottic carcinoma. Although a hoarse voice and odynophagia commonly occur after RT to the larynx, this is transient and rarely lasts longer than 6 weeks when using a short course (3–4 weeks) that is hyperfractionated.

22.   A. SLNB is recommended if staged T3N0.   This is false. At the time of writing, no consensus in the UK yet exists on the use of SLNB in head and neck cancer. No prospective randomized control trials currently exist comparing SLNB versus END for early oral cavity cancer. Guidance from the National Institute for Health and Care Excellence (NICE) updated in 2018 (NG36) recommends offering SLNB instead of END to people with early oral cavity cancer (T1–T2N0), unless they need cervical access at the same time such as for free-flap reconstruction. A meta-analysis by Yamauchi et al. (2015) pooled 987 patients and found a negative predictive value of 94%. Neck lymph node status is the single most important prognostic factor in HNSCC.

23.   C. N1 neck disease.   This is false. According to multidisciplinary guidelines for the management of oral cavity and lip cancer, adjuvant RT improves local control and overall survival when added to surgery in locally advanced cancers. It should be considered in all patients with either larger (T3 or T4) tumours and/or wherever there is ECS and/or in N2–3 neck disease. Other poor prognostic factors such as grade or perineural invasion may also inform the decision. Components of Broder's grading system are still used for describing oral SCC. Pattern of invasion and lymphoplasmacytic infiltrations are independent prognostic features of a poor outcome.

24.   A. If positive margins are found in the tongue excision, the patient should have chemotherapy or RT.   This is false. According to multidisciplinary guidelines for the management of neck metastases in head and neck cancer, SND alone is adequate treatment for pN1 neck disease without adverse histological features. Post-operative radiation or chemoradiation should be given for any patient with adverse histologic features following SND. However, if either ECS or positive margins are found then it should be chemoradiation. Age alone shouldn't preclude the use of chemotherapy in older adults with head and neck cancer.

25.   B. The posterior part of the submandibular triangle contains the external carotid artery.   Although nodes above the level of the hyoid bone are part of level II, if they lie medial to the carotid arteries then they are classed as retropharyngeal. Level III nodes radiologically are those anterior to the posterior edge of the SCM and lateral to the medial margin of the common carotid arteries. Level IVb nodes most often contain metastatic deposits from malignancies of the hypopharynx, subglottic larynx, trachea, thyroid, and cervical oesophagus. Oral cavity lesions drain most commonly to levels I–III and rarely to IVa. Level V is divided into a and b by the inferior edge of the cricoid cartilage.

26.   D. Nodal pathology should be confirmed by open surgical biopsy.   This is incorrect. Guidance from NICE updated in 2018 (NG36) recommends that nodal pathology should be confirmed by core biopsy, including testing for HPV and EBV. If PET–CT is negative then offer panendoscopy, targeted biopsies, and bilateral tonsillectomy. Tongue base mucosectomy is best performed using a robot.

27. D. Salvage surgical treatment should be offered. This patient has multiple comorbidities that significantly affect his prognosis, which combined with circumferential carotid involvement suggest incurable recurrence. Performance status is not a reliable substitute for comorbidity status as a prognostic measure. Triple therapy with platinum, cetuximab, and 5-FU appears to provide the best outcomes for the management of patients with recurrence who have a good performance status and minimal comorbidities. An SND is as effective as a modified radical neck dissection in this case. Patients with non-resectable recurrent disease should be offered the opportunity to participate in clinical trials of new therapeutic agents.

28. A. Surgical tracheostomy. Endoluminal debulking is instead preferred to tracheostomy. RT for painful bone metastases reports benefit in up to 50% of patients. Bisphosphonates improve pain control from bone metastases, but multidisciplinary guidelines state that they should only be given after RT and conventional pharmacology has been used.

29. A. Anaplastic thyroid carcinoma from thyroid lymphoma. This image shows the needle of a core biopsy, which is wider than those used in FNA. Both FNA and core biopsy are suitable for the diagnosis of papillary, follicular, medullary, and anaplastic thyroid carcinoma. Unlike FNA, core biopsy will help differentiate anaplastic thyroid cancer from thyroid lymphoma which can present in a similar manner.

30. D. Accessory. Sacrifice of the hypoglossal nerve (CN 12) will impair the motor supply to the intrinsic and extrinsic muscles of the tongue. Gaziano (2002) provides an excellent review of the evaluation and management of dysphagia in head and neck cancer. Swallowing deficits may result when any one or more of five cranial nerves are affected. The trigeminal nerve (CN 5) controls general sensation to the face and motor supply to the muscles of mastication. The facial nerve (CN 7) controls taste to the anterior two thirds of the tongue and motor function to the lips. The glossopharyngeal nerve (CN 9) provides general sensation to the posterior third of the tongue and motor function to the pharyngeal constrictors. The vagus nerve (CN 10) provides general sensation to the larynx and motor function to the soft palate, pharynx, larynx, and oesophagus.

References

Dey P, Arnold D, Wight R, MacKenzie K, Kelly C, Wilson J (2002). Radiotherapy versus open surgery versus endolaryngeal surgery (with or without laser) for early laryngeal squamous cell cancer. *Cochrane Database of Systematic Reviews* **2**:CD002027.

Gaziano JE (2002). Evaluation and management of oropharyngeal dysphagia in head and neck cancer. *Cancer Control* **9**(5):400–409.

Yamauchi K, Kogashiwa Y, Nakamura T, Moro Y, Nagafuji H, Kohno N (2015). Diagnostic evaluation of sentinel lymph node biopsy in early head and neck squamous cell carcinoma: a meta-analysis. *Head Neck* **37**(1):127–133.

Frerk C, Mitchell VS, McNarry AF, Mendonca C, Bhagrath R, Patel A, O'Sullivan EP, Woodall NM, Ahmad I (2015). Difficult Airway Society intubation guidelines working group. Difficult Airway Society 2015 guidelines for management of unanticipated difficult intubation in adults. *British Journal of Anaesthesia* **115**(6):827–848.

1. **A 14-year-old girl presents to your clinic after referral from an orthodontist. Her mother feels that her chin has started to deviate towards the patient's left side with a shift of her dental midline. She attributes it to a fall 4 years ago and shows you the scar on the right side of her chin. Which of the following is the single best answer?**

    A. Radiological examination will always demonstrate both horizontal and vertical enlargement of the condyle
    B. Radiological examination will demonstrate an old left condyle fracture
    C. Surgical treatment should be deferred until the patient is at least 18 years old
    D. 5 mm of deviation should be seen as an indication for surgical treatment
    E. A difference of 5% in bilateral condylar radioactive technetium uptake is significant

2. **You have harvested a non-vascularized cortical iliac crest graft but are awaiting the second team preparing the recipient site. Which of the following media are best for preservation of the most osteocytes in the graft?**

    A. 5% glucose solution wrapped in a swab refrigerated at 25°C
    B. Platelet poor plasma (PPP) in a pot uncovered at 25°C
    C. Normal saline in a pot uncovered at 25°C
    D. Normal saline soaked swab refrigerated at 4°C
    E. Wrapped in a dry swab refrigerated at 4°C

3. **Which of the following statements about the radiation dose for radiographs used in orthognathic practice is *false*?**

    A. A panoramic radiograph is approximately ten times the dose of a periapical
    B. The effective dose and not the absorbed dose is the most widely used comparator
    C. Younger patients are at greater risk than older patients
    D. The radiation doses produced by cone beam computed tomography (CBCT) machines are model dependent
    E. No evidence exists that a thyroid shield should be used routinely with CBCT radiographs

4. **A 10-year-old child presents with multiple carious teeth requiring extraction. His mother mentions that he snores a lot and is awaiting referral to the ear, nose, and throat team. His body mass index is 30. Which of the following is true?**
    A. The snoring will respond best to weight reduction
    B. In Crouzon syndrome snoring is due to mandibular hypoplasia
    C. First line surgical treatment is tonsillectomy with adenoidectomy
    D. This condition usually presents with daytime sleepiness
    E. The condition can be treated by a nasopharyngeal airway (NPA)

5. **Which of the following is false of the technique being utilized in Figure 3.1?**

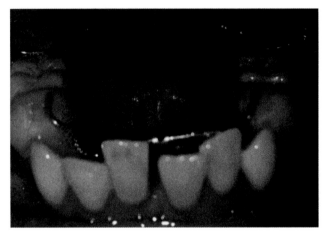

Figure 3.1 A device attached to the lower teeth.

    A. Orthodontics alone can be used prior to 8 years old until the suture fuses
    B. It is indicated for unilateral cross bite
    C. It is used to improve airway volume for obstructive sleep apnoea (OSA)
    D. Distraction should occur at a rate of 2 mm/day
    E. It is indicated for a unilateral scissor bite

6. **This patient has a mandible maxillary plane angle of 31 degrees. Which of the following is true of the procedure being performed?**
    A. The deformity could have potentially been treated with bucally placed anterior temporary anchorage device (TAD)
    B. This patient is set up in preparation for a bilateral posterior maxillary segmental osteotomy (PMSO)
    C. They will likely have a reduced lower anterior face height (LAFH)
    D. An indication for its use is a bilateral posterior scissor bite
    E. The patient is ready for surgery

7. **Sacrifice of which of the following arteries during planned maxillary downfracture reduces blood flow to the maxilla by 50%?**
    A. Posterior superior alveolar artery
    B. Infraorbital artery
    C. Descending palatine artery
    D. Ascending palatine branch of the facial artery
    E. Palatine branch of the ascending pharyngeal artery

8. **What is most true of the appliance being used in the clinical scenario shown in Figure 3.2?**

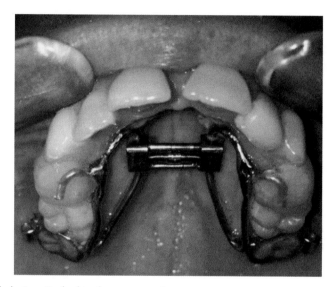

Figure 3.2 A device attached to the upper teeth.

    A. This patient must have reached skeletal maturity
    B. The degree of central incisor separation represents the degree of suture separation
    C. Posterior widening of the suture exceeds anterior widening
    D. Relapse rates of up to 10% occur
    E. It causes extrusion of the buccal molars

9. **The patient whose imaging is shown in Figure 3.3 is being investigated for progressive facial asymmetry. What is true of this imaging modality over its primary alternative?**
    A. It has slower image capture
    B. It uses a lower dose of radiation
    C. It utilizes technetium
    D. The images produced by it have worse spatial resolution
    E. It is safer for relatives to be around after the procedure

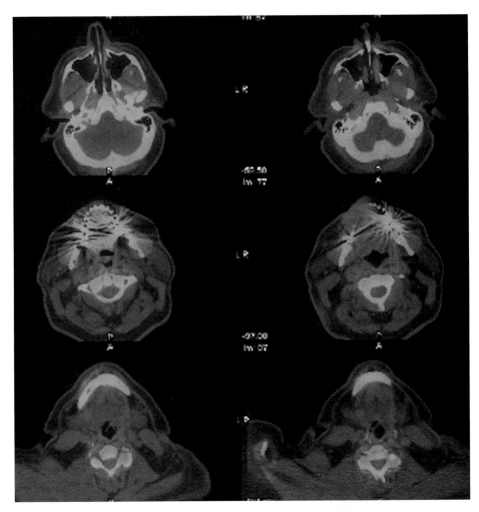

Figure 3.3 Cross-sectional imaging used.

10. **Which of the following features are specific for the condition shown in Figure 3.4?**
    A. Ramus displacement
    B. Midline deviation
    C. Inferior border concavity
    D. Condylar hyperplasia
    E. Canal displacement

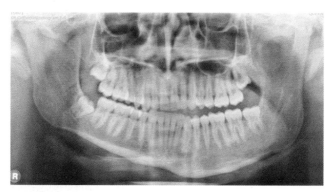

Figure 3.4 Orthopantomogram (OPG) of this patient on presentation.

11. Which is true of the modification of a maxillary osteotomy shown in Figure 3.5?

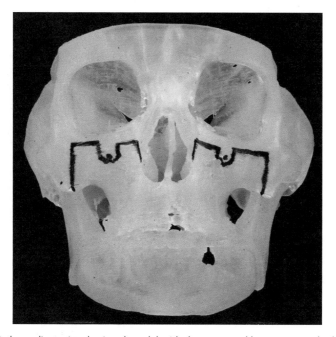

Figure 3.5 A three-dimensional printed model with the proposed bone cuts marked up.

    A. The incidence of relapse is higher than a conventional Le Fort I
    B. Iatrogenic nerve injury is higher than a conventional Le Fort I
    C. It is commonly called a Kuffner modification
    D. The lateral horizontal cuts are at the same level as a winged modification
    E. It is the only intraoral method for improving paranasal flattening

12. **A patient presents with an 8-mm anterior open bite (AOB) on a class 3 skeletal base. He has enlarged hands, feet, and tongue. Which sequence is most appropriate for treatment?**
   A. Reduction glossectomy then orthodontics then orthognathic surgery
   B. Reduction glossectomy then orthognathic surgery then orthodontics
   C. Orthognathic surgery combined with reduction glossectomy followed by orthodontics
   D. Orthodontics then reduction glossectomy then orthognathic surgery
   E. Orthodontics then orthognathic surgery then reduction glossectomy

13. **Regarding the Index of Orthognathic Functional Treatment Need (IOFTN):**
   A. It can apply to malocclusions amenable to orthodontic treatment alone
   B. Speech difficulties alone indicate a great need for treatment
   C. It does not apply to malocclusion following mandible fracture treatment
   D. Open bite equal or greater than 4 mm indicates a very great need for treatment
   E. It includes needs for treatment based upon degrees of crossbite

14. **What is true of the condition shown in Figure 3.6 the radiograph below that is causing a progressive facial asymmetry?**

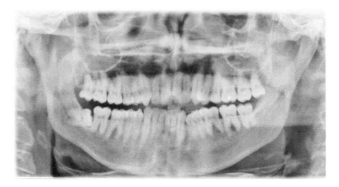

Figure 3.6 OPG of this patient on presentation.

   A. There is a relationship between scintigram uptake and specific histological findings
   B. It is due to an excess of insulin-like growth factor 1 (IGF-1)
   C. This is a type 1A deformity according to Wolford et al
   D. Left-sided crossbite would be expected
   E. Cartilage islands are pathognomonic for this condition

15. **During intraoral vertical ramus osteotomy, which of the following techniques are recommended for the proximal segment?**
    A. The lateral inferior muscular attachments should be stripped
    B. It should sit medial to the distal segment
    C. It should sit in line with the distal segment
    D. If it is overprojected then remove bone on its inferior surface
    E. Removal of bone prominences on its medial surface may be required

16. **A 15-year-old girl with ankylosing spondylitis presents with a class 2 occlusion and a mandibular midline shift of two incisor widths towards the affected side. Which is not part of an appropriate orthognathic surgery regime?**
    A. Unilateral alloplastic temporomandibular joint (TMJ) replacement
    B. Autologous fat packed around new joint
    C. Unilateral or bilateral coronoidectomy
    D. Clockwise mandibular advancement
    E. Concurrent maxillary osteotomy

17. **A 29-year-old with unilateral TMJ clicking and discomfort is being set up for a mandibular osteotomy. Which of the following images will be most predictive in anticipating future problems?**
    A. Soft tissue algorithm CT
    B. Hard tissue algorithm CT
    C. T1 weighted MRI
    D. T2 weighted MRI
    E. Single-photon emission computed tomography (SPECT)

18. **Which of the following surgical procedures used in the treatment of obstructive sleep apnoea (OSA) will *not* modify pharyngeal airway dimensions?**
    A. Maxillomandibular advancement (MMA)
    B. Turbinectomy
    C. Tonsillectomy
    D. Adenoidectomy
    E. Uvulopalatopharyngoplasty (UPPP)

19. **The highest level of evidence demonstrates which of the following associations between antibiotics and surgical site infections (SSIs) in orthognathic surgery?**
    A. Post-operative antibiotics reduce the risk of SSI compared to intrasurgical alone
    B. Short-term antibiotics are as good as long-term antibiotics
    C. The risk of side effects from long-term antibiotics outweighs their increased efficacy
    D. Short-term antibiotics reduce the risk of SSI relative to a single pre-operative dose
    E. Antibiotics reduce the incidence of subsequent non-union following SSI

20. **Which of the following surgical procedures would result in the least amount of post- operative orthodontics for the presentation shown in Figure 3.7?**

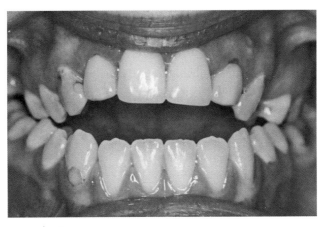

Figure 3.7 Anterior open bite on presentation.

    A. Le Fort I
    B. Surgically assisted rapid palatal expansion (SARPE)
    C. Two-part maxilla
    D. Three-part maxilla
    E. Four-part maxilla

21. **When comparing the post-operative stability of multi-part maxillary osteotomies, which of the following is true?**

    A. Maxillary widening is less stable than downpositioning
    B. Degree of surgical movement relates to stability
    C. SARPE produces less skeletal tipping than multi-part procedure
    D. Skeletal relapse exceeds dental relapse
    E. Instability is greater anteriorly than posteriorly

22. **Which of the following is false regarding the subsequent soft tissue changes following bone osteotomies?**

    A. In a maxillary setdown the upper lip lengthens by 50%
    B. In a three-part maxillary setback the upper lip moves by 50%
    C. In a chin augmentation the soft tissue pogonion moves by 80%
    D. In a mandibular setback the lower lip moves by approximately 90%
    E. In a maxillary advancement the nasal tip elevates by 50%

23. **A patient with a skeletal class 3 relationship presents with an AOB of 6 mm, increased LAFH, and spacing between the mandibular premolars bilaterally. What procedure are they likely to be having?**

A. Posterior segmental mandibular osteotomy

B. Kohle osteotomy

C. Anterior segmental mandibular osteotomy

D. Le Fort I osteotomy and posterior segmental mandibular osteotomy

E. Sowray–Haskell osteotomy

24. **Damage to which of the following cranial nerves is *not* a recognized complication of a maxillary osteotomy?**

A. 2

B. 3

C. 7

D. 10

E. 12

25. **A Caucasian 16-year-old girl presents to the joint orthognathic clinic following failed treatment with a twin block appliance. The ratio of LAFH to total anterior face height (TAFH) is 51%. The U1 to maxillary plane angle is 100 degrees. Which of the following is true?**

A. The treatment plan should include arch levelling

B. An aetiology of this presentation is lip hyperactivity

C. The overbite should be maintained prior to surgery

D. The nasolabial angle would be expected to be less than 90 degrees

E. Counterclockwise surgical mandibular rotation is required

1. D. 5 mm of deviation. Aesthetic studies have demonstrated that deviations less than 5 mm are not clinically visible. This patient most likely has condylar hyperplasia, which may have a vertical component, a horizontal component, or both. A blow to the left side of the chin may have caused damage to the left condylar head. However, as the occlusion was normal at the time, this would suggest that the fracture was minimally displaced and would likely have remodelled 3 years later. Hyperplastic growth can continue well into the mid-20s.

2. B. PPP in a pot uncovered at 25°C. Overall, studies have demonstrated that grafts stored in PPP have been found to preserve more osteocytes than saline or 5% dextrose solution. However, no studies demonstrated an improvement in outcome, and therefore saline-soaked gauze is still routinely used. Perioperative storage of cancellous bone under dry conditions should be avoided. Studies have reported no difference in cell viability after storage in saline for 4 hours at 4, 25, or 37°C.

3. E. No evidence exists that a thyroid shield should be used routinely with CBCT radiographs . There is evidence that thyroid shields are effective in reducing dose with large field of view (FOV) CBCT examinations. With limited FOV examinations the thyroid gland should be well away from the primary X-ray beam, but a thyroid shield should be used if available, and certainly for larger FOVs.

4. C. First line surgical treatment is tonsillectomy with adenoidectomy . This patient has OSA, of which the most common cause in children is enlarged adenoids and tonsils. However, surgery may involve removal of adenoids or tonsils and not necessarily both. There are differences between paediatric OSA and adult OSA. While adults usually have daytime sleepiness, children are more likely to have behavioural problems. NPAs are usually used in children less than 1 year old.

5. E. It is indicated for a unilateral scissor bite. This is a mandibular distraction device used to treat a transverse discrepancy, analogous to that used in a surgically assisted rapid maxillary expansion (SARME). A systematic review of mandibular midline distraction by de Gijt et al. demonstrated that this is most commonly used to treat severe mandibular crowding and bilateral mandibular crossbites. It has also been described for a unilateral scissor bite, reflecting the more severe skeletal discrepancy than a unilateral crossbite. The mandibular symphysis becomes fused at 1 year old and therefore functional appliances cannot be utilized to modify growth in the symphyseal area. There is no evidence to support maxillary–mandibular distraction improving airway volume and improvements are likely to be related to concurrent SARME procedures. Distraction should be undertaken at a similar rate to other distraction devices (generally 1 mm/day).

6. This patient is set up in preparation for a bilateral PMSO to treat a skeletal AOB. This is less commonly used than a posterior differential Le Fort I impaction. Posterior anchored

TADS in the palate can be used for smaller AOBs (no agreed cut-off exists, but 5 mm is often thought a maximum). Indications for PMSO include maxillary hyperplasia, distal replacement of the posterior maxillary alveolar fragment to provide space for proper eruption of an impacted canine, or a posterior crossbite or scissors bite. This patient is not yet ready for surgery as diastemas have not been created to enable space for the saw blade cuts.

7. C. Descending palatine artery. During downfracture of the maxilla, the nasopalatine and descending palatine arteries are invariably disrupted. The classic anatomical study undertaken by Bell et al. demonstrated that blood flow to the maxilla is reduced by 50% in the first post-operative day after sacrifice of the descending palatine arteries, but blood flow will eventually recover. The posterior superior alveolar and infraorbital arteries perfuse the maxillary buccal alveolus, periodontium, and teeth of the downfractured maxilla.

8. E. It causes extrusion of the buccal molars. This patient is undergoing transverse palatal expansion. This same device can be used for rapid maxillary expansion alone prior to approaching skeletal maturity, or with surgical assistance following that point. The opening of the midpalatine suture is non-parallel and triangular, with maximum opening at the incisor region and gradually diminishing towards the posterior part of the palate. The degree of separation between the central incisors should not be used as an indication of the amount of suture separation. There is buccal tipping and extrusion of the maxillary molars. Relapse rates of up to 30% occur.

9. E. It is safer for relatives to be around after the procedure. This patient has undergone a PET–CT scan with an 18F–sodium fluoride (18F–NaF) isotope. Compared to its main alternative (SPECT), PET–CT provides images with better spatial resolution and is quicker to perform (1.5 hours compared to 3.5 hours). The protein-bound fraction of radio-isotope is lower than a technetium one and the clearance from blood is faster.

10. E. Canal displacement. This patient has hemimandibular hyperplasia, a distinct clinical entity characterized by enlargement of the condyle, ramus, and mandibular body. The inferior convexity of the lower mandibular border and inferiorly displaced mandibular canal is also specific for diagnosis. The condyles in hemimandibular elongation (HE) are not hyperplastic. The term 'condylar hyperplasia' alone cannot be used to refer to hemimandibular hyperplasia (HH) or HE.

11. D. The lateral horizontal cuts are at the same level as a winged modification. This is a stepped modification of a Le Fort I maxillary osteotomy. It differs from a winged modification in that a vertical step is made both medially and laterally to the infraorbital nerve. A Kuffner is actually a modification of a Le Fort II osteotomy in that the cuts involve the infraorbital rim. A good summary of the Le Fort I modifications is provided by Catherine and Scolozzi (2019).

12. A. Reduction glossectomy then orthodontics then orthognathic surgery. This patient has an anterior open bite secondary to true macroglossia. It is challenging to perform orthodontics first in such cases as the tongue impedes movements and affects stability. Therefore reduction glossectomy is indicated prior to orthodontics, which is usually performed using an anterior resection combined with midline keyhole technique.

13. D. An open bite equal or greater than 4 mm indicates a very great need for treatment. First described by Ireland et al. in 2014, the IOFTN is increasingly being used in the UK to justify the need for orthognathic surgery in the National Health Service (NHS). Speech difficulties alone do not justify treatment. Skeletal abnormalities with occlusal disturbance as a result of trauma indicate a very great need for treatment. Scissor bites but not crossbites are included in the classification.

14. D. Left-sided crossbite would be expected. This patient has HE with excess horizontal growth of the condylar neck. Clinical features expected include a crossbite on the unaffected side and possibly a scissor bite on the affected side. It is a 1B deformity according to the classification described in Wolford et al. (2014) and is commonly used to build on that first described by Obwegeser and Makek. Cartilage 'islands' are pathognomonic for such excess condylar growth, but they can also be related to normal condylar growth. No clear association has been found between scintigram uptake and any specific histological findings. IGF-1 has been implicated, but causality has not been proven.

15. D. If it is overprojected then remove bone on its inferior surface. When handling the proximal segment during a Vertical Sub-Sigmoid Osteotomy (VSSO), the medial inferior muscular attachments should be stripped to prevent medial migration. The proximal segment should sit lateral to the distal segment to prevent upward rotation of the proximal segment and impingement of the inferior alveolar nerve. If the proximal segment feels overprojected, then 5 mm of bone should be removed from its inferior surface; this also reduces the chance of avascular necrosis. Removal of bone prominences on the inferior surface of the proximal segment may be required.

16. D. Clockwise mandibular advancement. This is not correct as the movement should be counterclockwise. This patient should have alloplastic TMJ replacement, which is normally performed at the same time as orthognathic surgery. Coronoidectomy is required if the rami are significantly advanced, as would have to be in this case.

17. C. T1 MRI. Wolford et al. (2003) investigated changes in TMJ dysfunction after orthognathic surgery, finding that of all the pre-operative variables, disc position was most indicative of future problems. In general, T1 MRIs are helpful in identifying disc position, alteration in bone and soft tissue structures, and interrelationships between bone and soft tissue anatomy. T2 MRIs are more helpful in identifying inflammatory responses in the TMJ.

18. B. Turbinectomy. The surgical treatment of OSA through MMA is occasionally performed in combination with additional procedures such as septoplasty, turbinectomy, tonsillectomy, adenoidectomy, UPPP, genial tubercle advancement, septoplasty, and turbinectomy. The latter two procedures do not modify pharyngeal airway dimensions.

19. A. Post-operative antibiotics reduce the risk of SSI compared to intrasurgical alone. A Cochrane Review in 2015 Brignardello-Petersen et al. by concluded from 11 studies that for people undergoing orthognathic surgery, long-term antibiotic prophylaxis decreases the risk of SSI compared with short-term antibiotic prophylaxis. This was still influenced strongly by the paper by Ruggles et al. from 1984. There is uncertainty whether short-term antibiotic prophylaxis decreases SSI risk relative to a single pre-operative dose of prophylactic antibiotics. There was no investigation of side effects of antibiotics in these 11 studies.

20. E. Four-part maxilla. The main indication of a four-piece maxilla is correction of a transverse maxillary deficiency which involves both the intercanine and intermolar width. It also allows differential vertical movements of the anterior and posterior segments of the maxilla.

21. A. Maxillary widening is less stable than downpositioning. Studies identifying the stability of segmental osteotomies are heterogeneous, but some broad conclusions can be made. Dental relapse exceeds skeletal relapse for both SARPE and three- piece osteotomies. Maxillary widening with three-part segmentation is the least stable procedure of all orthognathic surgeries. SARPE produces more skeletal tipping than the multi-part procedure.

22. E. In a maxillary advancement the nasal tip elevates by 50%. In fact, in a widely quoted doctoral thesis, Soncul demonstrated that in maxillary advancement the nasal tip elevates by 30%.

23. B. Kohle procedure. This procedure comprises an anterior segmental osteotomy in conjunction with a genioplasty. It enables correction of an open bite as well as vertical genioplasty in one surgical appointment.

24. C. 7. Damages to cranial nerves 2, 3, 4, 6, 10, and 12 have all been reported during maxillary osteotomies, due to fracture propagation through the skull base. Facial nerve damage during mandibular ramus osteotomies is reported with an incidence of 0.5–1%.

25. B. An aetiology of this presentation is lip hyperactivity. The Eastman normal value for LAFH/TAFH in a Caucasian population is 55%, with a standard deviation of 2%. An aetiology of this presentation is hyperactive or hypertonic lips. The nasolabial angle would be expected to be obtuse. In skeletal class 2 cases, particularly with a class II division 2 incisal relationship (108 degrees +/− 5 degrees) and reduced vertical dimensions, the lower arch should not be levelled completely prior to surgery. Instead a curve of Spee should be maintained in the lower archwire to facilitate a three-point landing.

References

Bell WH, You ZH, Finn RA, Fields T (1995). Wound healing after multisegmental Le Fort I osteotomy and transection of the descending palatine vessels. *Journal of Oral and Maxillofacial Surgery* **53**:1425–1433.

Brignardello-Petersen R, Carrasco-Labra A, Araya I, Yanine N, Cordova Jara L, Villanueva J (2015). Antibiotic prophylaxis for preventing infectious complications in orthognathic surgery. *Cochrane Database of Systematic Reviews* Issue 1. Art. No.: CD010266. doi:10.1002/14651858.CD010266.pub2. Accessed 25 January 2022.

Catherine Z, Scolozzi P (2019). Modified Le Fort I step osteotomy for improvement of paranasal flatness in maxillary deficiency: Technical note and series of 24 cases. *Journal of Oral and Maxillofacial Surgery* **120**(6):559–565. doi:10.1016/j.jormas.2019.07.003. Epub 2019 Jul 9. PMID: 31299342.

de Gijt JP, Vervoorn K, Wolvius EB, Van der Wal KG, Koudstaal MJ (2012). Mandibular midline distraction: a systematic review. *Journal of Cranio-Maxillofacial Surgery* **40**(3):248–260. doi:10.1016/j.jcms.2011.04.016. Epub 2011 Jun 29. PMID: 21719302.

Ireland AJ, Cunningham SJ, Petrie A, Cobourne MT, Acharya P, Sandy JR, Hunt NP (2014). An index of orthognathic functional treatment need (IOFTN). *Journal of Orthodontics* **41**(2):77–83. doi:10.1179/1465313314Y.0000000100. PMID: 24951095; PMCID: PMC4063315.

Obwegeser HL, Makek MS. (1986). Hemimandibular hyperplasia—hemimandibular elongation. *Journal of Oral and Maxillofacial Surgery* **14**(4):183–208. doi:10.1016/s0301-0503(86)80290-9. PMID: 3461097.

Ruggles JE, Hann JR (1984). Antibiotic prophylaxis in intraoral orthognathic surgery. *Journal of Oral and Maxillofacial Surgery* **42**(12):797–801.

Soncul M, Bamber MA (2004). Evaluation of facial soft tissue changes with optical surface scan after surgical correction of Class III deformities. *Journal of Oral and Maxillofacial Surgery* **62**(11):1331–1340. doi:10.1016/j.joms.2004.04.019. PMID: 15510353.

Wolford LM, Reiche-Fischel O, Mehra P (2003). Changes in temporomandibular joint dysfunction after orthognathic surgery. *Journal of Oral and Maxillofacial Surgery* **61**(6):655–660; discussion 661. doi:10.1053/joms.2003.50131. PMID: 12796870.

Wolford LM, Morales-Ryan CA, García-Morales P, Perez D (2009). Surgical management of mandibular condylar hyperplasia type 1. *Proceedings (Baylor University, Medical Center)* **22**(4):321–329. doi:10.1080/08998280.2009.11928546. PMID: 19865502; PMCID: PMC2760163.

1. **A patient has had a wide local excision of a presumed basal cell carcinoma (BCC) from the right forehead. This demonstrates a melanoma with a Breslow thickness of 1.7 mm with ulceration that has been narrowly excised. What is the next most appropriate management step?**
   A. Wide local excision with a 1-cm margin and dressing pending further histology
   B. Wide local excision with a 1-cm margin and reconstruction as appropriate
   C. Wide local excision with a 2-cm margin and reconstruction as appropriate
   D. Wide local excision with a 1-cm margin, reconstruction, and sentinel lymph node biopsy
   E. Wide local excision with a 2-cm margin, reconstruction, and sentinel lymph node biopsy

2. **A 74-year-old man who is a renal transplant recipient attends with an exophytic lesion on the scalp measuring 5 cm in diameter. Excision is performed down to the periosteum with split thickness skin graft, and histology reveals a poorly differentiated squamous cell carcinoma (SCC) with a close (0.2–mm-deep) margin. The split thickness graft has failed. What is the most appropriate next step?**
   A. Watchful waiting and regular dressings to encourage granulation
   B. Removal of the outer table of the calvarium and application of a dermal matrix substitute
   C. Removal of the outer table of the calvarium and reconstruction with free tissue transfer
   D. Adjuvant radiotherapy
   E. Adjuvant treatment with intravenous cemiplimab

3. **A 48-year-old woman presents with a pigmented lesion on her cheek that demonstrates areas of depigmentation and a blue-white veil on dermoscopy. What is the most likely diagnosis?**
   A. Pigmented BCC
   B. Morphoeic BCC
   C. Solar lentigo
   D. Lentigo maligna
   E. Melanoma

4. **A 56-year-old man has an excision biopsy demonstrating a BRAF wild-type melanoma from the left forehead (Breslow 1.7 mm, ulcerated). He goes on to have a wide local excision and sentinel node biopsy, which shows one positive sentinel node with a subcapsular deposit measuring <0.1 mm. What is the next most appropriate step?**
    A. Close clinical follow-up
    B. A completion lymph node dissection (CLND)
    C. Adjuvant radiotherapy
    D. Adjuvant treatment with nivolumab
    E. Adjuvant treatment with dabrafenib and trametinib

5. **A 55-year-old fit and healthy woman presents with a nodular lesion on her right nasal ala. Biopsy confirms a micronodular BCC. What is the most appropriate management?**
    A. Wide excision and immediate reconstruction
    B. Wide excision and delayed reconstruction pending histology
    C. Mohs micrographic surgery (MMS) and reconstruction
    D. Cryotherapy
    E. Topical 5-fluorouracil

6. **A 60-year-old man presents with a nodular lesion clinically and dermoscopically consistent with a BCC on the dorsum of the nose. This is excised and reconstructed with a glabellar flap repair. Histology demonstrates a nodular BCC excised with a 3.8-mm-deep margin and 2.3-mm peripheral margin but surrounding superficial BCC extending to the peripheral margin at 3 o'clock (involved). What is the appropriate further management?**
    A. Further wide local excision and delayed reconstruction pending histology
    B. MMS
    C. Topical 5-fluorouracil therapy
    D. Cryotherapy
    E. Topical imiquimod

7. **A 65-year-old woman has a lesion, which is clinically suspicious of a SCC of the lower lip measuring <2 cm. What is the most appropriate next step in management?**
    A. Wide local excision and direct closure
    B. Staging computed tomography (CT) scan of the neck and thorax
    C. Ultrasound (US) +/– fine needle aspiration cytology (FNAC)
    D. Wide local excision and Abbe–Estlander flap
    E. Magnetic resonance imaging (MRI) of the neck

8. **An exophytic lesion is excised from the lower lip of a 45-year-old smoker and found to be a poorly differentiated SCC with perineural invasion in a nerve >0.1mm diameter excised with a peripheral margin of 4.8 mm and deep margin of 12.1 mm. What is the next most appropriate step?**

   A. Further wide local excision and reconstruction as appropriate

   B. Close clinical follow-up

   C. Staging CT scan of the neck and thorax

   D. Adjuvant radiotherapy

   E. Adjuvant chemotherapy with cemiplimab

9. **A 78-year-old man is scheduled for a wide excision of a 4-mm nodule from the helix of the right pinna. A helical advancement flap is planned. The patient is on dabigatran for atrial fibrillation. The patient's estimated glomerular filtration rate is >90 ml/min/1.73 m². What is the most appropriate course of action?**

   A. Withhold dabigatran for 24 hours prior to surgery

   B. Withhold dabigatran for 36 hours prior to surgery

   C. Withhold dabigatran for 48 hours prior to surgery

   D. Withhold dabigatran for 72 hours prior to surgery

   E. Do not withhold dabigatran prior to surgery and continue as normal

10. **An 86-year-old man has a biopsy of an exophytic lesion on his scalp, which suggests an atypical fibroxanthoma (AFX). He undergoes a wide local excision and subsequently histology demonstrates a pleomorphic dermal sarcoma (PDS) excised by 8 mm peripherally and 1.7 mm deep (taken to the periosteum and repaired with a split thickness skin graft). What is the next most appropriate management step?**

    A. Staging CT scan of the neck, thorax, abdomen, and pelvis

    B. Wide excision with a 2-cm margin and reconstruction as appropriate

    C. Adjuvant radiotherapy

    D. Sentinel node biopsy

    E. Watchful waiting

11. **A 30-year-old man presents with a 2-cm-diameter fixed red-brown nodule on his neck strongly suspected of being a dermatofibrosarcoma protuberans (DFSP) based on clinical appearances. What would the recommended treatment be?**

    A. Wide local excision +/– reconstruction as appropriate with a 1-cm margin

    B. Wide local excision +/– reconstruction as appropriate with a 2-cm margin

    C. MMS

    D. Radiotherapy

    E. Chemotherapy with imatinib mesylate

12. A 45-year-old woman has a wide local excision of a non-ulcerated 1.3-mm Breslow thickness melanoma from the left pinna and refuses sentinel node biopsy. At a follow-up within the first year she is noted to have a lymph node in level II and FNAC demonstrates malignant melanoma, with no other nodes seen on cross-sectional imaging and no distant metastases (stage IIIB). What is the next step?

A. Immunotherapy with ipilimumab and nivolumab
B. Radical radiotherapy
C. Parotidectomy and level II–V therapeutic neck dissection
D. Level I–V therapeutic neck dissection
E. Level II–V therapeutic neck dissection

13. A 57-year-old man undergoes a wide local excision and sentinel lymph node biopsy for a stage IIA (T2bN0M0) nodular melanoma from the right posterior neck. This is confirmed to be a BRAF wild-type. The sentinel lymph node shows no tumour deposits. At a further follow-up in the first year he develops three subcutaneous pigmented nodules between the wide local excision scar and the right axilla. Further imaging confirms no lymphadenopathy or distant metastases. What is the next step in treatment?

A. Immunotherapy
B. Cryotherapy of the nodules
C. Conservative excision of the nodules
D. Wide excision of the nodules and repeat sentinel lymph node biopsy
E. Electrochemotherapy of the nodules

14. Which of the following dressings would you choose for a heavily exuding wound following failure of a full thickness skin graft?

A. Allevyn®
B. Tegaderm™
C. Actiform Cool®
D. Mepitel®
E. Granuflex®

15. A 37-year-old woman presents with a 12-mm-diameter lentiginous macule on the left cheek. A small incisional biopsy reveals appearances in keeping with a lentigo melanoma. What is the most appropriate management?

A. Topical imiquimod
B. Excision with a narrow margin (2-mm) and primary closure
C. Excision with a 5-mm margin and local flap repair
D. Excision with a 5-mm margin and delayed repair pending histology
E. Excision with a 1-cm margin and local flap repair

16. **A 45-year-old woman has a biopsy of a non-healing ulcer on her nasal tip. Histology demonstrates an infiltrative BCC. She undergoes MMS leaving her with a defect encompassing 65% of her nasal tip with preservation of the lower lateral cartilage. Given high cosmetic expectations, what is your reconstructive method of choice?**

   A. Paramedian forehead flap to the existing defect
   B. Removal of the remainder of the nasal tip and reconstruction with a paramedian forehead flap
   C. Full thickness skin graft
   D. Removal of the remainder of the nasal tip and insertion of a full thickness skin graft
   E. Bilobed flap

17. **A 64-year-old woman undergoes MMS for a BCC of the lower lid, resulting in a full thickness defect of greater than 2/3 of the horizontal width. What would be the reconstructive technique of choice?**

   A. Direct closure
   B. Lateral canthotomy and cantholysis to facilitate closure
   C. Tenzel flap
   D. Modified Hughes tarsoconjunctival flap
   E. Cutler–Beard flap

18. **You intend to lengthen a 10-mm scar by a further 5 mm that is distorting the angle of the mouth. At what approximate angle would you make the incision in relation to the long axis of the scar?**

   A. 30 degrees
   B. 45 degrees
   C. 60 degrees
   D. 75 degrees
   E. 90 degrees

19. **Review of the histology of a 6-mm infiltrative BCC of the nasal alar demonstrates incomplete excision at the deep margin but complete peripherally. Reconstruction was with a nasolabial pedicled flap. The patient has dementia and resides in a nursing home but is co-operative with treatment. What is the recommended management?**

   A. Surveillance is preferable, considering the patient's co-morbidities
   B. There is a 70–100% chance that re-excision will demonstrate residual tumour
   C. Radiotherapy is the preferable treatment option
   D. A deep re-excision margin of 4–5 mm is recommended
   E. Further peripheral re-excision at the inferior margin should be performed

20. **A patient presents with an 18-mm lesion on the forehead. Biopsy demonstrates nodular BCC. The patient does not want surgical excision. The least appropriate treatment option would be:**
   A. Topical imiquimod
   B. Cryosurgery
   C. Photodynamic therapy
   D. Cautery with curretage
   E. Radiotherapy

21. **Which of the following common terms used in pathology reports to describe histological alterations in skin structure are true?**
   A. Acanthosis is hypoplasia of the epithelium
   B. Papillomatosis is the formation of a papilloma in the epidermis
   C. Hyperkeratosis is an increase in the number of keratinocytes in the stratum lucidum
   D. Parakeratosis is the presence of nucleated cells at the skin surface
   E. Keratosis is an increase in the size of keratinocytes in the epidermis

22. **A patient presents with a 24-mm SCC of the lower lip centred on the midline affecting the skin and mucosa. Which of the following lip reconstruction techniques is the *least* likely to induce microstomia?**
   A. Abbe
   B. Estlander
   C. Gillies
   D. Webster–Bernard
   E. Karapandzic

23. **Which of the following suture techniques used in skin closure will achieve the maximal skin eversion?**
   A. Simple interrupted suture
   B. Vertical mattress suture
   C. Horizontal mattress suture
   D. Subcuticular suture
   E. Running locking suture

24. **Which of the following is true of dermatoscopy?**
   A. It enhances surface reflections to maximize details from the epidermis and dermis
   B. Both non-polarized and polarized types are commonly utilized
   C. Contact fluid is always required for function
   D. Melanin in the dermis will appear black
   E. It improves diagnostic accuracy in detecting malignancy by untrained clinicians

25. Which of the following malignant lesions are *not* appropriate to treat with cryosurgery in clinic for a frail nursing-home resident who is not fit for surgery?

A. Morpheaform BCC

B. SCC in situ

C. Lentigo maligna melanoma

D. Superficial BCC

E. Keratoacanthoma

1. E. Wide local excision with a 2-cm margin, reconstruction, and sentinel lymph node biopsy. Evidence would support a margin of 2 cm (anatomy permitting) based on the Breslow thickness. As a stage IIA according to the American Joint Committee on Cancer (AJCC) 8th edition, a sentinel node would be recommended to offer valuable prognostic information and determine the need for completion lymph node dissection.

2. B. Removal of the outer table of the calvarium and application of a dermal matrix substitute. Surgical re-excision of the close margin would be recommended to ensure adequate clearance. Some multidisciplinary teams (MDTs) would recommend formal outer table excision following splitting of the calvarium and others would recommend burring of the outer table. His age and co-morbidities would make free tissue transfer a less desirable option where a simpler reconstructive option might be permissible. There are good precedents in the literature for the use of dermal matrix substitutes such as Integra® for full thickness scalp defects.

3. E. Melanoma. The blue-white veil is indicative of dermal involvement and the lesion having a depth suggestive of a breach in the basement membrane. This coupled with the areas of depigmentation in a pigmented lesion would make melanoma the most likely diagnosis and certainly warrant an excisional biopsy.

4. A. Close clinical follow-up. The risk of non-sentinel lymph node (NSLN) positivity has been worked out with various nomograms, but the Dewar criteria and Rotterdam criteria are the most widely used, based on the pattern of deposits in the sentinel node and tumour burden, respectively. With such a small tumour burden in the least worrying configuration (subcapsular), an argument could be made for the risks outweighing the benefits of completion dissection, even for a high-risk site (head and neck).

5. C. MMS and reconstruction. The high-risk site coupled with the need to keep the defect as small as possible whilst still oncologically safe demands MMS. There are limited reconstructive options and realistically one would want the superior clearance achieved with the smallest possible defect created.

6. C. Topical 5-fluorouracil therapy. As the residual tumour is superficial and a local flap has been used in reconstruction, it would be acceptable in this instance to treat the superficial component topically with chemotherapy.

7. A. Wide local excision and direct closure. Lip SCCs are treated as cutaneous malignancies rather than head and neck mucosal malignancies. As such, in the absence of clinically detectable lymphadenopathy, staging scans are generally not required. Clearly, surgical excision is the mainstay of treatment, and given the size of the lesion, excision with an adequate margin is still likely to be amenable to a wedge excision rather than an Abbe–Estlander flap.

8.   D. Adjuvant radiotherapy.   Perineural invasion is a marker of heightened risk for recurrence, and MDT recommendation would almost certainly be for adjuvant radiotherapy, unless there are compelling reasons to the contrary. As this is a cutaneous malignancy, you only do cross-sectional imaging of the neck if there are clinically palpable nodes.

9.   E. Do not withhold dabigatran prior to surgery and continue as normal.   Guidance such as that issued by the British Society of Dermatological Surgery (BSDS) (2016) would recommend continuation of novel oral anticoagulants for what is perceived to be a moderate risk procedure.

10.   A. Staging CT scan of the neck, thorax, abdomen, and pelvis.   The distinction between AFX and PDS cannot be made often on the basis of a biopsy alone and requires formal excision. Wider margins of 1–2 cm are recommended to provide for this eventuality of the diagnosis of a PDS, and in this event, staging scans are required at the outset, along with referral to a specialist skin cancer multidisciplinary team (SSMDT) and/or sarcoma MDT, depending on local protocol.

11.   C. MMS.   Mohs surgery for head and neck DFSPs has been shown to result in lower recurrence rates and where available would be recommended following discussion with an SSMDT. An excellent reference paper for these and other cutaneous adnexal tumours is provided by Green et al. (2015).

12.   C. Parotidectomy and level II–V therapeutic neck dissection.   The paper by Newlands and Gurney (2014) is an excellent resource for discussion of an evidence-based approach to surgery for nodal basin involvement in head and neck melanoma. This is stage IIIB disease that is surgically resectable and as such immunotherapy would not have a place in primary management. Radiotherapy has no place as a primary treatment modality, but the role for adjuvant radiotherapy is explored in the presentation of the results of the TROG trial by Burmeister et al. (2012).

13.   C. Conservative excision of the nodules.   In the absence of regional lymphadenopathy and distant metastases, the management of in-transit disease is symptomatic largely. For some sites cryotherapy may be in order, particularly when there are multiple nodules that would render surgery difficult or unduly painful. For a small number of nodules, surgical excision is an acceptable treatment modality. In the limbs, the option of isolated limb infusion is available for widespread in-transit disease.

14.   A. Allevyn®.   It is worth knowing some common dressing types, including proprietary names and broad categories. For heavily exudative wounds, an absorbent foam dressing is recommended.

15.   D. Excision with a 5-mm margin and delayed repair pending histology.   In this instance, excision is with the recommended margin for a lentigo maligna (5 mm) but enabling further wider margins pending definitive histology of the entire specimen. It is possible that there is an invasive component that is yet to be sampled and that the biopsy has not been representational, in which case a wider margin based on Breslow thickness +/− sentinel node may be warranted.

16.   B. Removal of the remainder of the nasal tip and reconstruction with a paramedian forehead flap.   The gold standard of nasal reconstruction is the paramedian forehead flap in terms of skin colour match and quality. Unless this encroaches close to the rim, support grafts should not be required if the lower lateral cartilages are preserved. The general rule is that if over 50% of a subunit is removed, the remainder of the subunit should be sacrificed to optimize the cosmetic outcome.

17. D. Modified Hughes tarsoconjunctival flap.   Given the horizontal discrepancy and the need for reconstruction of the posterior lamella as well as the anterior lamella, a Hughes flap is required, in combination with either a lateral advancement flap (e.g. Mustarde) or a skin graft (e.g. contralateral upper eyelid). An alternative reconstructive option might be an oral mucosal graft along with a bipedicled Triper flap from the upper lid. The Cutler–Beard flap is used in reconstruction of the upper lid. A Tenzel flap would not address the posterior lamellar and is only good for shorter defects.

18. B. 45 degrees.   In this particular case you are aiming to increase the length of the scar by 50%, which approximately equates to a 45-degree angle. Other generalized increases in length include 25% (30 degrees), 75% (60 degrees), and 100% (75 degrees).

19. E. Further peripheral re-excision at the inferior margin should be performed. Studies are surprisingly heterogenous and re-excision of incompletely excised lesions reports the presence of residual tumour in 30–50% of cases. Adequate surveillance would realistically be highly challenging in such a patient. Peripheral excision margins for recurrent BCC of 5–10 mm have been suggested, but no such recommendations exist for deep margin involvement. Although no peripheral involvement was found, standard histological examination may have missed some involvement and most clinicians would undertake further peripheral excision unless it would compromise the functional result.

20. B. Cryosurgery.   Photodynamic therapy can be used for primary superficial and nodular BCC. To date, there is no good evidence to support its use for infiltrative or recurrent BCC. Cryosurgery is on occasion used for low-risk BCCs but has the lowest evidence base of these options to support it.

21. D. Parakeratosis is the presence of nucleated cells at the skin surface.   Acanthosis is hyperplasia of the epithelium. Papillomatosis is an increase in the depth of the corrugations at the junction between the epidermis and dermis. Hyperkeratosis involves a thickening of the stratum corneum layer. The stratum lucidum comprises layers of dead, flattened keratinocytes. Parakeratosis is the presence of nucleated cells at the skin surface. Keratosis is a generic clinical description of thickening of the skin used with conditions such as frictional keratosis and is not a strict histological term.

22. D. Webster–Bernard.   This flap is used to reconstruct the lower lip by advancing cheek tissue and the remaining lip tissue medially. This technique is best suited for subtotal defects of the lower lip where the commissure is preserved. Cheek skin is recruited to add length to the lip repair to lessen the degree of microstomia.

23. C. Horizontal mattress suture.   The horizontal mattress suture is useful for wounds under high tension because it provides wound eversion and strength, because it spreads tension along a wound edge. It is commonly used for pulling wound edges together over a distance or as the initial suture to anchor two wound edges (often termed holding sutures).

24. B. Both non-polarized and polarized types are commonly utilized.
A dermatoscope eliminates surface reflections to reveal details from the epidermis and upper layers of the dermis. Newer dermatoscopes allow non-contact dermoscopy by employing polarizing lenses that negate the need for a contact fluid. There are few differences in terms of indications

between non-polarized and polarized types. Colour recognition is important in dermatoscopy, with the identification of melanin in different layers being key. Melanin appears black when very superficial, but deeper in the epidermis it appears brown, and in the dermis appears either grey or blue. Dermoscopy improves diagnostic accuracy among trained specialists, but when used by untrained clinicians it is likely no better than visual inspection.

25.   A. Morpheaform BCC.   Although both BCC and SCC can be treated with cryosurgery, it is usually reserved for the superficial variants of BCC and SCC in situ. However, current guidelines do not recommend cryosurgery for morpheaform BCC. The lentigo maligna variant of melanoma can be treated effectively due to its superficial nature and sensitivity of melanocytes to freezing.

References

British Society for Dermatological Surgery (2016). *Guidance on Antithrombotics and Skin Surgery, August 2016*. London: BSDS. https://bsds2020.wpengine.com/wp-content/uploads/2020/10/bsds-guidance-on-antithrombotics-and-skin-surgery-august-2016.pdf.

Burmeister BH, Henderson MA, Ainslie J, et al (2012). Adjuvant radiotherapy versus observation alone for patients at risk of lymph node field relapse after therapeutic lymphadenectomy for melanoma: a randomized trial. *Lancet Oncology* **13**:589–597.

Green B, Godden D, Brennan A (2015). Malignant cutaneous adnexal tumours of the head and neck: an update on management. *British Journal of Oral and Maxillofacial Surgery* **53**:485–490.

Newlands C, Gurney B (2014). Management of regional metastatic disease in head and neck cutaneous malignancy: 2. Cutaneous malignant melanoma. *British Journal of Oral and Maxillofacial Surgery* **52**:301–307.

1. **A 65-year-old man sustained an isolated zygomatic arch fracture which was treated as a day case by a Gilles lift. He has recently been started on ramipril for long-standing hypertension. The following day the patient presents to the emergency department with a temporal swelling. Which of the following is the most likely cause for the swelling?**
    A. Submasseteric space infection
    B. Sialocele
    C. Superficial temporal space collection
    D. Deep temporal space infection
    E. Overcorrection of fracture reduction

2. **A 24-year-old patient with a penetrating neck injury and ongoing bleeding is being taken to theatre. Computed tomography (CT) scan demonstrates a vascular flush associated with the common carotid artery. Their heart rate is 110 beats per minute and respiratory rate 24 breaths per minute. The anaesthetist notices that the pulse pressure is reducing. Which of the following is most likely to be taking place?**
    A. Blood loss of 750 ml
    B. Reduced diastolic pressure
    C. Class II shock
    D. Class III shock
    E. Peri-arrest

3. **You are asked by the on-call team to review a 34-year-old patient with a traumatic head injury and difficulty with speech. CT scan demonstrates a coronoid fracture of the mandible. Which one of the following is true of a coronoid fracture of the mandible?**
    A. More common than fractures of the ramus
    B. Tends to be displaced
    C. Always requires treatment if displaced
    D. Results in trismus
    E. Should be treated intra-orally

4. **CT scan demonstrates an isolated mandibular condyle fracture with a malocclusion. Which of the following is an absolute indication for open reduction internal fixation (ORIF) of the condylar head?**

    A. Vertical displacement of 8 mm
    B. Bilateral condyle fractures
    C. Malocclusion
    D. Lateral extracapsular displacement
    E. Gross comminution of the condylar head

5. **A patient has been booked into trauma clinic following a suspected nasal fracture. The patient was injected with local anaesthetic in the emergency department for a procedure, yet their nose still appears deviated. Potential sequelae had this not been performed include all but one of the following?**

    A. Saddle nose
    B. Septal perforation
    C. Septal destruction
    D. Cavernous sinus thrombosis
    E. Nasal tip necrosis

6. **A 57-year-old woman taking clopidogrel for a recent myocardial infarction has sustained a fractured angle of the mandible. Indications to extract the third molar in the fracture line in the first 48 hours post injury include all but one of the following?**

    A. Tooth fracture
    B. Pre-existing pericoronal infection
    C. Pre-existing periapical infection
    D. Interference with fracture reduction
    E. Interference with plate position

7. **You are called to see a patient on the ward who is 2 hours following alloplastic repair of an orbital floor fracture. Visual acuity has been measured as 6/36 and heart rate is 100 beats per minute. Which of the following interventions should be undertaken first?**

    A. Remove suture
    B. Administer acetozalimide
    C. Administer analgesia
    D. Administer steroids
    E. Record visual acuity

8. You are called to the emergency department to review a patient
    involved in a road traffic accident. The patient is in pain, has
    blurred vision, and has diplopia in all ranges of movement. CT scan
    demonstrates a sphenoid bone fracture. Which of the following is true?

    A. They will have a relative afferent pupillary defect
    B. Damage is likely due to fracture of the frontal bone
    C. There will likely be enophthmos from the orbital wall injury
    D. Ptosis and mihydriasis will be present
    E. Cheek numbness will be present

9. You are asked to review the facial fractures of an intubated patient in
    the intensive care unit. Their nasal tip appears to be upturned and their
    intercanthal distance is 36 mm. There is gross comminution of the
    lacrimal crests including the tendinous insertion. Which of the following
    is true?

    A. The interpupillary distance would be expected to be over 60 mm
    B. The palpebral fissure will be lengthened
    C. Transnasal canthopexy through a coronal approach alone is sufficient
    D. Assessment should include an inferior distraction test
    E. Formal assessment of the lacrimal duct should be deferred until after surgery

10. Which of the following statements regarding complications of mandible
    fractures is false?

    A. In malunion, the mandible fracture heals by fibrous union with segments in non-anatomic
        position, leading to altered function
    B. Non-union of the fracture may result from gross bone loss, interposition of non-osseous
        material, or inadequate immobilization
    C. Delayed union is uncommon in facial fractures but may be caused by inadequate
        immobilization of the fracture, infection, or malnutrition
    D. Fat embolism may complicate fracture
    E. Avascular necrosis may complicate comminuted fractures but is rare in the head and
        neck region

11. You are called to review a patient in the emergency department with
    a grossly displaced orbital roof fracture noted on a head CT scan taken
    20 minutes ago. The patient gets double vision when they attempt to
    look at the corner of their mouth but gets increasingly confused when
    you attempt to assess other eye movements. Which of the following
    is true?

    A. Urgent neurosurgical review is required
    B. Superior oblique muscle is likely damaged
    C. Inferior oblique muscle is likely entrapped
    D. Superior rectus is likely entrapped
    E. Repeat head CT scan is indicated

12. **A 5-year-old child involved in a road traffic accident presents with a fractured mandibular parasymphysis and condylar neck. Which of the following statements is true?**

    A. Closed reduction is contraindicated in this age group
    B. Open reduction must use resorbable methods of osteosynthesis
    C. Conservative treatment will reduce the chances of ankylosis
    D. Open reduction should be attempted if the condylar head is dislocated out of the glenoid fossa
    E. A buccal acrylic splint is appropriate if the fractures are mildly displaced

13. **A family has been involved in a road traffic collision. Both the 10-year-old child and her grandmother require suturing of similar facial lacerations. Which of the following are true?**

    A. The child will have a better cosmetic result than her grandmother
    B. Deeper sutures are more important for the grandmother's lacerations than the child's
    C. At 6 months the scars will be more prominent in the child
    D. At 6 months the scars will be wider in the child
    E. Vitamin supplementation is likely to be beneficial to both patients

14. **A 20-year-old patient presents to the emergency department with pain and ecchymosis around one eye. CT scan demonstrates a 2-day-old isolated fracture of the orbital floor. Their visual acuity is reduced and blood is seen covering the iris, which dissipates upon laying the patient flat. Which of the following is false?**

    A. The pain is likely due to soft tissue injury
    B. Urgent intra-ocular pressure measurement is required
    C. The patient should be sat up to at least 45 degrees
    D. The patient requires the medical treatment that is utilized in the management of retrobulbar haemorrhage
    E. This may represent major underlying intraocular trauma

15. **Which of the following is true of this method of fracture fixation shown in Figure 5.1?**

    A. It is suitable for comminuted fractures
    B. A countersinking tool is used to create a platform in the far cortex
    C. The screw should be inserted perpendicular to Champey lines
    D. The technique requires lag screws to work
    E. Drill the near cortex to the external diameter of the screw

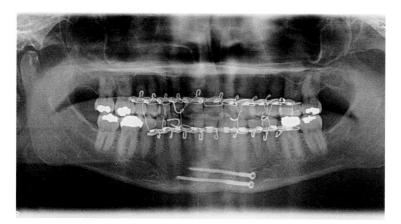

Figure 5.1 OPG radiograph showing previous fixation of a mandible fracture.

16. **You are about to operate on an 8-year-old boy on the emergency list who was attacked by a dog the previous afternoon. He has been too traumatized for the wound to be fully examined, but a photograph provided by his mother clearly shows some tissue dangling off his cheek. He is allergic to penicillin. Which of the following is true?**
    A. Wounds closed primarily within 12 hours do not require prophylactic antibiotics
    B. A course of oral clindamycin is recommended post-operatively
    C. You should obtain consent from his parents for a local flap
    D. The dangling piece of tissue should be excised prior to closure
    E. A 20% infection rate is to be expected despite antibiotics if closed primarily

17. **The patient shown in Figure 5.2 is 16 days post injury. Gross comminution is seen on CT scan, with a 10-mm missing segment just above the glabellar. Which of the following techniques in repair will optimize the aesthetic outcome?**
    A. Undertaking the repair as quickly as possible
    B. Ensuring contact between all bone ends is <5 mm
    C. Use of a collagen injectable filler
    D. Polyether ether ketone (PEEK) implant placement through an endoscopic approach
    E. Hydroxyapatite cement injected percutaneously

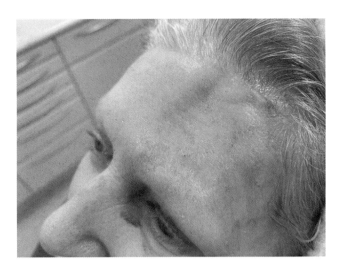

Figure 5.2 Gross indentation of the left side of the forehead seen clinically.

18. **A 29-year-old patient underwent repair of a mandible fracture 3 months prior. They are now unable to move their lip downwards or evert. Electromyography (EMG) demonstrates no evidence of depressor activity. Which of the following is recommended?**
    A. Cross facial nerve graft
    B. Anterior belly of digastric transfer
    C. Microsurgical transfer of extensor digitorum brevis
    D. Extensor labii brevis resection
    E. Botulinum toxin injection of contralateral depressors

19. **Which of the following muscles is preferential in surgical rehabilitation of the post-traumatic injury shown in Figure 5.3 in terms of minimizing iatrogenic side effects from reconstruction?**
    A. Buccinator
    B. Anterior belly of digastric
    C. Genioglossus
    D. Hypoglossal
    E. Zygomaticus major

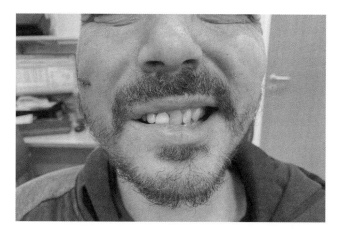

Figure 5.3 Facial weakness seen post injury.

20. **A 22-year-old man presents to the emergency department with a penetrating neck wound. Despite extensive packing placed pre-hospital there is on-going blood loss, which is estimated to be 1.5 litres so far. This patient is likely to:**
    A. Be hypotensive and bradycardic
    B. Have reduced production of inflammatory mediators including cytokines and oxidants
    C. Be coagulopathic due to dilution of clotting factors
    D. Have a renal blood flow of 1.5 litres per minute
    E. Have microcirculatory hypoxia caused by vasoconstriction

21. **The patient shown in Figure 5.4 is 7 days following treatment of facial injuries. Which one of the following treatment modalities is not recommended?**
    A. Scopolamine
    B. Aspiration
    C. Botulinum toxin
    D. Ductal repair
    E. Propantheline bromide

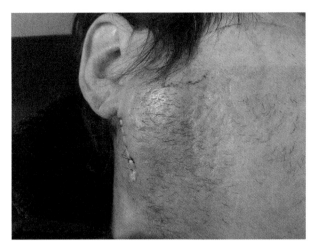

Figure 5.4 Right-sided pre-auricular swelling.

22. What is true of the clinical scenario shown in Figure 5.5?

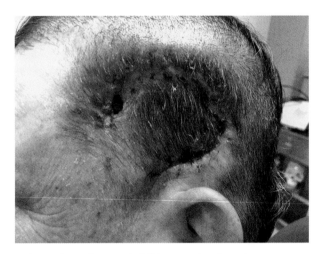

Figure 5.5 Depression and scarring seen in left temporal scalp region.

    A. The original pathology was most likely a stroke
    B. The flap design was appropriate
    C. Cranioplasty should be performed
    D. Vacuum assistance closure dressing is indicated
    E. Bone will be present in the abdomen

23. The patient in Figure 5.6 is being treated for pan facial fractures. In what scenario is this airway most likely to be appropriate?

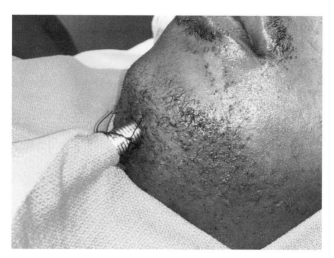

Figure 5.6 Intra-operative intubation during trauma surgery.

    A. Limited mouth opening
    B. Polytrauma
    C. Severe head injury
    D. Haemoglobin count <80
    E. BMI >40

24. The patient in Figure 5.7 sustained an avulsive defect of their whole scalp. Reanastomosis of the superficial temporal arteries failed after 72 hours and this dressing was placed. Which of the following is true?

    A. Pericranium must have been present for this technique to work
    B. A dermal substitute such as Integra® cannot be used with this technique
    C. The scalp should be shaved before anastomosis is attempted
    D. An underlying bone defect would not have been present
    E. The choice of anastomosis is primarily determined by vessel caliber

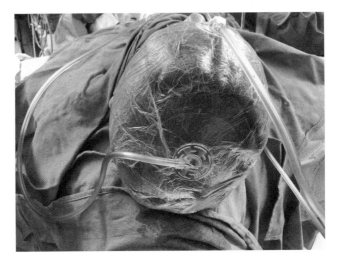

Figure 5.7 Treatment of an avulsive defect of the whole scalp.

25. **The patient shown in Figure 5.8 presents 24 hours after receiving a blow to the face. He is complaining of double vision on upwards gaze. There is a large step at both the left infra-orbital rim and left frontozygomatic suture. The left pupil fails to dilate when a light is shone into it. Which of the following is true?**

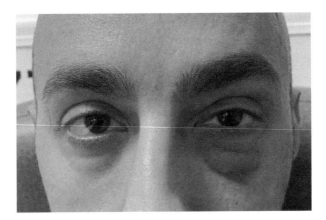

Figure 5.8 Clinical appearance following facial trauma to the patient's left side.

A. A Naugle exophthalmometer is likely to assist in clinical assessment
B. Diplopia on upward gaze demonstrates that the inferior rectus muscle is trapped
C. Alteration in cheek sensation is helpful in making the diagnosis
D. A fixed dilated pupil suggests that the patient has a concomitant head injury
E. A Hertel exophthalmometer is of little use at this stage in management

26. **The patient with this CT scan (Figure 5.9) is awaiting surgery. No orbital floor defect is seen. What is true of treating this fracture?**

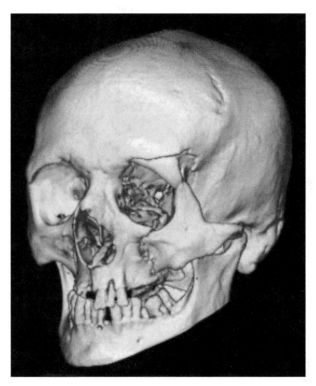

Figure 5.9 CT scan of the left zygomatic complex.

    A. Local incisions alone are appropriate
    B. The sphenozygomatic suture will assist in intra-operative reduction
    C. Reduction is guided by symmetry of the malar prominences
    D. Orbital exploration is necessary to prevent complications
    E. Diplopia on upward gaze is likely

27. **The patient shown in Figure 5.10 had treatment of her mandibular condyle fracture 3 weeks ago. What is the most appropriate next step in management?**

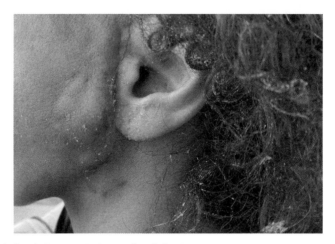

Figure 5.10 Left-sided pre-auricular swelling following surgery.

A. Surgery
B. Archbars
C. Aspiration
D. Antibiotics
E. Botulinum toxin

28. **You are called by the emergency department consultant regarding a patient injured in an explosion at work when standing immediately next to a gas cylinder. A metallic object has been noted on the chest CT scan shown in Figure 5.11. The patient is dysphonic with oxygen saturation of 92% on air. There is some venous oozing from a wound in the neck. Which of the following management options should be undertaken first?**

A. Blood administration
B. Intubation
C. Surgery
D. CT scan
E. Cervical (C) spine stabilization

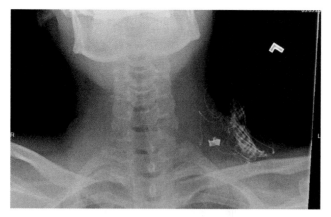

Figure 5.11 Plain radiograph of the neck in a trauma patient.

29. **The patient shown in Figure 5.12 returns 5 days following treatment of a mandibular body fracture. Part of the top plate is visible. The occlusion is unchanged and there is no mobility. They have just completed a course of post-operative antibiotics. The most appropriate management option would be:**

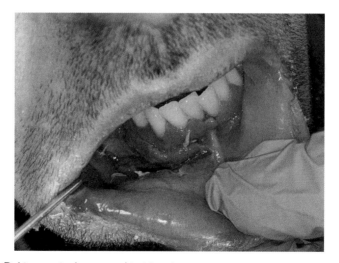

Figure 5.12 Dehiscence in the mucosal incision site.

A. Repeat surgery via an intra-oral approach
B. Reassurance
C. Repeat antibiotics
D. Suturing
E. Repeat surgery via a transcutaneous approach

30. The patient in Figure 5.13 was attacked with a machete. Most of the wound edges lie lower on one side than the other and some edges are longer than others. Which technique will not optimize the aesthetic result?

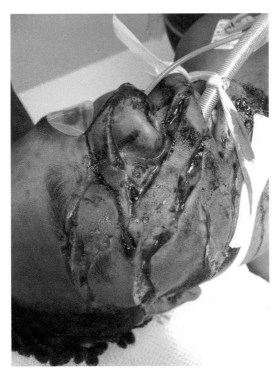

Figure 5.13 Complex facial lacerations.

    A. The suture should be passed more superficially on the long side and deeper on the short side

    B. In cross-section, deep suture passage should be triangular-shaped, with its base located deeply

    C. The skin edges should always be everted when suturing is complete

    D. The suture should be passed more superficially on the low side and deeper on the high side

    E. The dermal suture should enter the deep reticular dermis on the incised edge of the wound

1. C. Superficial temporal space collection. The zygomatic arch borders the superficial temporal space. A collection may develop within hours of treatment, but an infection would be rare and would be seen after a few days. Angiotensin converting enzyme (ACE) inhibitors can cause generalized facial swelling.

2. D. Class III shock. Class I and II haemorrhagic shocks do not display hypotension. This decrease in pulse pressure is primarily related to a rise in the diastolic component due to an increase in circulating catecholamines which increase the vascular tone and resistance. Systolic pressure changes minimally in early haemorrhagic shock.

3. E. Should be treated intra-orally. Coronoid fractures are very uncommon. They are rarely displaced as they are splinted by the action of temporalis. They should be treated by an intra-oral approach if they cause limitation in lateral excursions.

4. D. Lateral extracapsular displacement. Lateral extracapsular displacement remains a widely accepted indication for surgery and was first described by Zide and Kent. The prospective trial described by Eckelt et al. (2006) added indications such as shortening of the ramus by 2 mm and a fragment angulation of greater than 10 degrees.

5. E. Nasal tip necrosis. Potential sequelae of infected septal haematoma are saddle nose, septal perforation, septal destruction, or cavernous sinus thrombosis (via the emissary vein). It does not cause nasal tip necrosis.

6. E. Interference with plate position. Although patients on clopidogrel are at increased risk of intra-operative bleeding, there is no indication to delay treatment for the 5 days that would be required to reduce serum levels to that similar of a normal patient. Interference with reduction is an indication for tooth removal. Monocortical fixation is not reliant upon tooth position at the angle of the mandible.

7. B. Acetozalimide. This patient has reduced visual acuity and likely tachycardia due to pain. Such a post-operative patient should be suspected to have retrobulbar haemorrhage. Immediate treatment is to return to the operating theatre. The decision is assisted by accurate recording of visual acuity which should demonstrate a progressive deterioration. Acetazolamide has no role in acute management in this scenario.

8. D. Ptosis and mihydriasis will be present. This patient has superior orbital fissure (SOF) syndrome, with the fissure lying between the lesser and greater wings of the sphenoid bone. SOF manifests as ptosis, ophthalmoplegia (causing diplopia), and exophthalmos. SOF causes forehead numbness but not cheek numbness, which is due to damage to the infra-orbital nerve, which travels through the infra-orbital fissure. Blindness or reduced visual ability may manifest as a relative afferent pupillary defect, representing additional injury to the optic nerve which results in orbital apex syndrome.

9. E. Formal assessment of the lacrimal duct.   This patient likely has traumatic telecanthus from an untreated naso-ethmoidal fracture. According to the Markowitz–Manson scoring system this is a type 3 fracture, which is generally treated by transnasal canthopexy or reattachment of the canthus to the lacrimal bone followed by reduction if required; both require a coronal flap with lower eyelid incision.

10.   A. In malunion, the mandible fracture heals by fibrous union with segments in non-anatomic position, leading to altered function.   In a malunion of a mandible fracture, normal osseous healing occurs, but the segments are not in the optimal anatomical position. The true incidence of malunion is not known as only a small proportion of mandible fractures are ever left to heal in a non-optimal position. Those fractures without an adequately functioning occlusion are generally re-operated on early before a malunion can occur.

11.   A. Urgent neurosurgical review is required.   Superior oblique palsy is a complication of closed head trauma. The depressing action of the superior oblique muscle makes the eye look down towards the mouth). The superior oblique muscle itself is incredibly rarely damaged, even with damage to the orbital roof.

12.   D. Open reduction should be attempted if the condylar head is dislocated out of the glenoid fossa.   Paediatric mandibular fractures are rare, with the vast majority treated conservatively. Closed reduction is most commonly performed using acrylic splints. It is, however, possible to apply interdental wire fixation or even Erich arch bars to primary teeth. Although even the most severely damaged condylar head fractures will likely remodel, displacement outside of the glenoid fossa will likely result in ankylosis and subsequent facial growth alteration.

13.   B. Deeper sutures are more important for the grandmother's lacerations than the child's.   Aged patients have slower wound healing and less wound contraction. The decreased tensile strength in particular means that wounds are more likely to open up if placed under tension. Aged patients, however, get less scarring, and any scars may be less prominent in relation to relaxed skin tension lines. Vitamin C and zinc are essential to enable cells to multiply and multivitamin supplementation is recommended in patients who are potentially nutritionally deficient.

14.   D. Requires the medical treatment that would be utilized in retrobulbar haemorrhage.   Hyphema is defined as the presence of blood within the aqueous fluid of the anterior chamber. The most common cause of hyphema is blunt trauma, and even when small it may represent major underlying intraocular trauma. Treatment is with topical agents, with systemic carbonic anydrase inhibitors and hyperosmotic agents (acetazolamide or mannitol) only required if this fails to control the pressure.

15.   E. Drill the near cortex to the external diameter of the screw.   Because lag screw technique compresses the fracture fragments together, the use of this technique is contraindicated in comminuted fractures, and in addition, the screw must be placed perpendicular to the fracture plane. This image uses lag screws, but the technique can be modified slightly to enable screws without a smooth proximal head to be used. A countersinking tool is used to create a platform in the near cortex. An excellent description of this technique is shown on the AO website.

16. A. Wounds closed primarily within 12 hours do not require prophylactic antibiotics. Guy and Zook back in 1986 reported a wound infection rate of 1.4% following primary closure of 145 head and neck dog bite wounds without administration of antibiotics, and this study is frequently cited as the basis for the recommendation not to use prophylactic antibiotics in the primary treatment of these injuries. Avulsive tissue defects from dog bites are surprisingly rare. Only minimal trimming of wound edges is indicated because facial tissue can survive on small pedicles. Clindamycin is recommended for penicillin-allergic patients, but wounds closed primarily within 12 hours do not require prophylactic antibiotics. Antibiotic prophylaxis is also advocated for orocutaneous bite wounds of the cheek, because of their additional exposure to the victim's own oral flora.

17. B. Ensuring contact between all bone ends is <5 mm. This patient has sustained a comminuted fracture of the frontal bone. Repair between 2 and 8 weeks post injury is not recommended as the neo-osteogenesis will render bony reduction more difficult, and persistent soft tissue swelling may prohibit satisfactory recontouring. Gaps less than 5 mm are unlikely to be noticeable. On balance, filler injections for defects that extend into the glabellar region are not recommended due to the risk of unilateral vision loss. Both methyl methacrylate and hydroxyapatite cement require an open approach for application. These materials are not suitable for the repair of full-thickness anterior table defects.

18. E. Botulinum toxin injection of contralateral depressors. This patient has sustained injury to their marginal mandibular nerve, causing paralysis of depressor anguli oris and depressor labii muscles. For injuries less than 12 months, and with EMG evidence of depressor activity, Terzis et al. has demonstrated the best option is by direct neurotization of depressors using a cross facial nerve graft. If longer than 12 months, use a hypoglossal nerve transfer, but again depressor activity is required. Depressor labii brevis resection has been used successfully but effectively prevents further alternative treatments being performed in the future.

19. B. Anterior belly of digastric. This patient has weakness of the buccal and marginal mandibular branches of the facial nerve. The anterior belly of the digastric muscle receives innervation from the inferior alveolar nerve and can be transferred and used during correction of paralysis involving the marginal mandibular branch of the facial (VII) nerve. Although the hypoglossal (XII) nerve can also be used in reconstruction in a patient with facial paralysis, altered tongue mobility is an adverse effect. The buccinator and zygomaticus major muscles receive sensory innervation from the facial nerve, as does the posterior belly of the digastric muscle. These muscles would not be effective in ipsilateral reconstruction for facial paralysis. The genioglossus muscle, supplied by the hypoglossal nerve, is located in the tongue. Tongue muscle cannot be transferred for reconstruction.

20. E. Have microcirculatory hypoxia caused by vasoconstriction. Loss of 1.5 litres is equivalent to 20–30% of blood volume. Stimulation of the sympathetic nervous system causes a peripheral vasoconstriction and tachycardia. Bradycardia does not occur until 40% of circulating blood volume has been lost. Bleeding leads to poor tissue perfusion that induces an inflammatory response characteristic of ischaemic-reperfusion injury, with increased production of cytokines and oxidants. In this scenario, no intravenous fluids have been administered and so there is no dilution and no coagulopathy. 1.5 litres per minute is an increased rate and in fact blood flow would be reduced as it is diverted away from non-vital organs.

21. D. Ductal repair.   This patient has a sialocele secondary to treatment of a condyle fracture using a transparotid approach. Glandular sialoceles such as this generally resolve with conservative measures such as serial aspiration supplemented by topical (scopolamine/hyoscine) or systemic (propantheline) anticholinergics.

22. D. Vacuum assistance closure dressing is indicated.   This patient has had a classic reverse question-mark incision used for a decompressive craniectomy. This is most likely required for a traumatic brain injury. In this case the flap was too small, likely compromising the superficial temporal artery. A cranioplasty can only be inserted if the wound bed is healthy. Subcutaneous preservation of the autologous bone flap in the abdomen has largely been abandoned due to perceived concerns of resorption.

23. E. BMI >40.   A tracheostomy should be chosen over a submental intubation if prolonged intubation is required (such as a severe head injury), multiple visits to theatre are expected (polytrauma), mouth opening is limited (tube changing is difficult), or an increased chance of intra-operative bleeding is expected.

24. C. The scalp should be shaved before anastomosis is attempted.   This patient is undergoing topical negative pressure wound therapy. The choice of vessel for anastomosis is more determined by vessel damage than caliber. It is important to carefully examine the scalp for damage prior to anastomosis and shaving of the hair is recommended.

25. E. A Hertel exophthalmometer is of little use at this stage in management.
The patient likely has a left zygomatico-orbital fracture resulting in enophthalmos. A fixed dilated pupil in the trauma setting is more likely to be traumatic mydriasis. A Naugle exophthalmometer is a superior and inferior orbital rim-based instrument and therefore requires the rim to be non-displaced. Similarly, the Hertel requires both frontozygomatic sutures to be intact.

26. E. Diplopia on upward gaze is likely.   Should the patient desire treatment, this presentation will require a bicoronal flap to access the supraorbital fracture in addition to vestibular and lower eyelid incisions. Judging reduction using the symmetry of malar prominences is rarely helpful and certainly of no use if three fracture sites are being openly reduced. The fracture of the rim is overlapped, which in conjunction with the lack of floor defect makes impingement of the inferior rectus likely.

27. A. Surgery.   This patient has had ORIF of the condyle through a transcutaneous approach. She failed to comply with a soft diet and the plate has bent and the screws have become loose. This appearance is of an abscess and not a sialocele. Infection in this area is highly unlikely to heal with antibiotics alone and at 3 weeks it would be best to remove the metalwork.

28. B. Intubation.   This patient likely has blast lung (primary blast) based upon the clinical findings with a related history of exposure within close proximity to an explosive detonation. The energized fragment (secondary blast) is highly unlikely to be responsible for such symptoms. A blast lung has reduced compliance and in this case would likely necessitate mechanical ventilation following intubation. Dysphonia and venous oozing are soft signs of penetrating neck injury that do not warrant early exploration.

29. C. Repeat antibiotics. Intra-oral wound dehiscence generally heals with continued antibiotics alone, even when a load sharing plate is partially exposed, as long as the fracture is stable and has not moved.

30. D. The suture should be passed more superficially on the low side and deeper on the high side. All of the other four techniques would in this scenario evert the wound edges, thereby optimizing the aesthetic result. If one of the wound edges lies lower than the other, the suture should be passed through the cut edge of the skin low on that side ('low-on-the-low').

References

AO Surgery Reference Guide. Accessed at: https://surgeryreference.aofoundation.org/cmf/trauma on 25 Jan 2021.

Eckelt U, Schneider M, Erasmus F, Gerlach KL, Kuhlisch E, Loukota R, Rasse M, Schubert J, Terheyden H (2006). Open versus closed treatment of fractures of the mandibular condylar process-a prospective randomized multi-centre study. *Journal of Cranio-Maxillofacial Surgery* **34**(5):306–314.

Guy RJ, Zook EG (1986). Successful treatment of acute head and neck dog bite wounds without antibiotics. *Annals of Plastic Surgery* **17**(1):45–48. doi:10.1097/00000637-198607000-00009. PMID: 3078618.

Terzis JK, Tzafetta K (2009). "Babysitter" procedure with concomitant muscle transfer in facial paralysis. *Plastic and Reconstructive Surgery* **124**(4):1142–1156. doi:10.1097/PRS.0b013e3181b2b8bc. PMID: 19935298.

Zide MF, Kent JN (1983). Indications for open reduction of mandibular condyle fractures. *Journal of Oral and Maxillofacial Surgery* **41**(2):89–98. doi:10.1016/0278-2391(83)90214-8. PMID: 6571887.

1. **A 94-year-old man presents with bilateral slow-growing parotid gland enlargement. Ultrasound reveals two well-circumscribed hypoechogenic masses in each parotid gland, with cytology from fine needle aspirate of the largest lesion in the right parotid suggestive of either Warthin's tumour or pleomorphic adenoma. What is the most appropriate management?**
   A. Serial review with ultrasound
   B. Open parotid biopsy
   C. Right superficial parotidectomy
   D. Bilateral superficial parotidectomy
   E. Core biopsy of the right parotid gland lesion

2. **A 57-year-old Afro-Caribbean woman presents with recurrent obstruction of her right submandibular gland. Investigations reveal a 9-mm-diameter sialolith at the hilum of the gland, which is palpable on clinical examination. What is the most appropriate management?**
   A. Removal of the submandibular gland
   B. Sialendoscopy and Dormia® basket retrieval
   C. Sialendoscopy and Stonebreaker™ pneumatic lithotripter
   D. Intra-oral hilar dissection
   E. Extracorporeal shockwave lithotripsy

3. **A 17-year-old girl presents with multiple confluent papules in the nasolabial folds that on excision have proved to be trichoepitheliomas. She has multiple lumps on her scalp that have proved to be cylindromas on excision. She now presents with a mobile lump in the left parotid. What is the most likely histopathological diagnosis on superficial parotidectomy?**

   A. Basal cell adenoma
   B. Mucoepidermoid carcinoma
   C. Pleomorphic adenoma
   D. Warthin's tumour (adenolymphoma)
   E. Adenoid cystic carcinoma

4. **A 42-year-old woman with Sjögren's syndrome complains of bilateral parotid swelling and pain. Ultrasonographic appearances suggest multiple hypoechoic solid nodules bilaterally and evidence of intraparenchymal obstruction. What is the next step in management?**

   A. Serial clinical review with ultrasonography
   B. Intraglandular botulinum toxin
   C. Sialendoscopy with intraductal steroid
   D. Open parotid biopsy
   E. Ultrasound-guided fine needle aspiration biopsy

5. **Which of the following is not an indication for consideration of adjuvant radiotherapy following removal of a malignant salivary gland tumour?**

   A. T2 tumour
   B. Close surgical margin
   C. Involved surgical margin
   D. Perineural invasion
   E. Positive ipsilateral neck nodes (pN+) on histology

6. **A 24-year-old man complains of a persistent dry mouth for over 3 months. Which of the following would not be contributory to the diagnosis of primary Sjögren's syndrome?**

   A. Labial salivary gland biopsy with focal lymphocytic sialadenitis and focus score of >/= 1 foci/4 mm^2
   B. Anti-SS-A/Ro positive
   C. Anti-SS-B/La positive
   D. Schirmer's test </= 5 mm/5 minutes in at least one eye
   E. Unstimulated whole saliva flow rate </= 0.1 ml/minute

7. **A 36-year-old woman has a dry mouth and eyes persisting for more than 3 months. An autoantibody screen is positive for anti-SS-A/Ro antibodies and a labial gland biopsy demonstrates focal lymphocytic sialadenitis. Which of the following co-morbidities would preclude a diagnosis of primary Sjögren's syndrome?**
   A. Active hepatitis B infection
   B. Active hepatitis C infection
   C. Human immunodeficiency virus (HIV) positivity on antiretroviral therapy
   D. Previous pulmonary tuberculosis
   E. Lyme disease

8. **A 55-year-old woman with a past medical history of autoimmune pancreatitis presents with bilateral painless parotid enlargement and an accompanying dry mouth. A magnetic resonance imaging (MRI) scan shows diffuse symmetrical enlargement of both parotid glands but no masses, with low T2 signal intensity. An open biopsy demonstrates storiform fibrosis and lymphoplasmocytic infiltrate. Which further investigation would be most helpful?**
   A. Ultrasound
   B. Sialography
   C. Sialendoscopy
   D. Serum immunoglobulin G4 (IgG4)
   E. Anti-SS-A/Ro antibodies

9. **A patient who had a Warthin's tumour excised from their left parotid gland 4 years ago has developed what is likely one on their left side. They had persistent Frey's syndrome that was resistant to Botox® following the first operation. What would be an appropriate treatment modality?**
   A. Prophylactic topical anticholinergics
   B. No modification is required
   C. Rotation of a tempoparietal fascia flap
   D. Raising a thick skin flap
   E. Prophylactic botulinum type A injections

10. **A 58-year-old patient presents with the slow growing lump shown in Figure 6.1 under their tongue for the last 2 months. Excisional biopsy demonstrates pseudocystic changes with epithelioid macrophages forming the periphery but with a small area of marked atypia centrally. What is the next most appropriate step?**
    A. MRI scan of the head and neck
    B. Repeat excisional biopsy
    C. Sialogram
    D. Surveillance
    E. Bleomycin injection

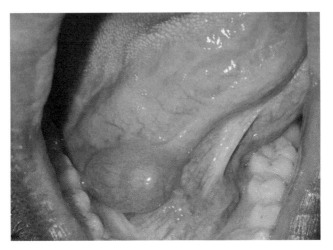

Figure 6.1 Lump under the tongue.

11. **A 60-year-old woman with rheumatoid arthritis presents with an enlarging pre-auricular mass over 6 months. What origin will the cells of the mass likely be?**
    A. Myoepithelial
    B. Epithelial
    C. Lymphocyte
    D. Osteoblast
    E. Adipocyte

12. **A patient presents with a long-standing pre-auricular lump that has recently increased rapidly in size. The histology from a core biopsy demonstrates serous and myoepithelial cells but with keratin deposition. Imaging of the head and neck region demonstrates an isolated parotid lesion with no other pathology. Which of the following is true?**
    A. Imaging of this lesion will demonstrate a well-defined margin
    B. Extraparotid infiltration of this lesion is rare
    C. The lesion originates from the parotid gland
    D. Facial nerve involvement from this lesion is unlikely
    E. This lesion is associated with a good long-term prognosis

13. **A symptomatic patient demonstrates the imaging shown in Figure 6.2. They wish to have the treatment with the lowest complication rates. Which of the following modalities would you recommend?**

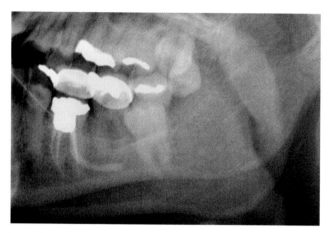

Figure 6.2 Radiograph of a symptomatic patient undergoing investigation.

   A. Intracorporeal lithotripsy
   B. Extracorporeal lithotripsy
   C. Intraluminal basket retrieval
   D. Intra-oral excision
   E. Gland excision

14. **A 15-mm mass is identified on CT scan in the supra-hyoid region. The relationships of the mass include the styloid process posteriorly, the superior constrictor muscle medially, and the angle of the mandible laterally. Which of the following is true of the mass?**
   A. It lies within the carotid space
   B. It is most likely an adenoid cystic carcinoma
   C. Fine needle aspiration biopsy of the mass is contraindicated
   D. It will likely be symptomatic
   E. A neurilemoma should be suspected

15. **A fit and well 62-year-old presents with three small pre-auricular lumps at the site of a parotid tumour excised 15 years previously. Which of the following modalities is the *least* preferable management option?**
   A. Surveillance
   B. Nerve sparing surgery
   C. Radiotherapy
   D. Nerve sparing surgery + radiotherapy
   E. Nerve sacrifice surgery + radiotherapy

1. A. Serial review with ultrasound. The multifocality and bilaterality support the idea of a Warthin's tumour or adenolymphoma. Given the patient's age, in the absence of symptoms, conservative management would be the recommended management.

2. D. Intra-oral hilar dissection. The stone is too large and proximal for sialendoscopy, and in most practices this would automatically translate to a sialadenectomy due to the limited availability, complications, and guarded success rates of lithotripsy. Combes et al. (2009) presents a technique of intra-oral hilar dissection with compelling results which should form part of the mainstay of modern salivary gland management.

3. A. Basal cell adenoma. The picture fits with a diagnosis of Brooke–Spiegler syndrome and the salivary gland tumours tend to be basal cell adenomas rather than other subtypes in the context of the syndrome. The confluence of paranasal trichoepitheliomas, scalp cylindromas, and salivary gland disease is a strong indicator of this rare condition, caused by mutations in the CYLD gene. This is a purposeful example of an 'off the wall' question sometimes present in the examination based on rare entities seen by examiners; as long as nobody can't answer it, as you'll see from the standard setting chapter it won't be excluded!

4. D. Open parotid biopsy. With a background of Sjögren's syndrome, the symptoms are suggestive of intraparenchymal obstruction secondary to inflammation. This may be amenable to steroids (and intraductal washout with rituximab has also been suggested). The priority at the outset, however, is an open biopsy of the parotid tail to exclude a low-grade mucosa-associated lymphoid tissue (MALT) lymphoma.

5. A. T2 tumour. The evidence base for adjuvant radiotherapy in salivary gland tumours suffers from heterogeneity of patient populations and follow-up periods. There are no randomized controlled data, but there have been some large cohort studies (e.g. Piedbois et al. 1989; Armstrong et al; 1990; Terhaard et al; 2005). Generally, adjuvant radiotherapy shows improved local control in the event of T3/T4 tumours, close margins, involved margins, bone invasion, perineural invasion, and/or pN+ neck.

6. C. Anti-SS-B/La positive. The diagnosis of primary Sjögren's syndrome is made based on clinical features in combination with weighting of all of the above with the exception of anti-SS-B/La antibodies. It also includes an ocular staining score of >/=5 or van Bijsterveld score of >/= 4 according to the American College of Rheumatology/European Alliance of Associations for Rheumatology (ACR/EULAR) classification criteria.

7. B. Active hepatitis C infection. In the ACR/EULAR criteria, the following are exclusion criteria for the diagnosis of primary Sjögren's syndrome: a history of head and neck radiation; active hepatitis C infection; acquired immunodeficiency syndrome (AIDS); sarcoidosis; amyloidosis; graft-versus-host disease; IgG4-related disease.

8. D. Serum IgG4. The clinical picture, imaging findings, and histology are in keeping with Mikulicz's disease, an IgG4-related disease with raised serum levels of IgG4 being diagnostic. The associated pancreatitis and storiform fibrosis are strong clues. Treatment is with corticosteroids, with the addition of steroid-sparing immunosuppressants where required.

9. B. No modification is required. Several surgical techniques have been described for preventing Frey's, of which the most common are shown in the list of possible answers, in addition to a sternocleidomastoid flap and a superficial musculoaponeurotic system (SMAS) flap. All have disadvantages, and for routine excision of a Warthin's tumour, even if the patient had Frey's before, none would be indicated. Medical treatment is not given prophylactically.

10. A. MR scan of head and neck. This patient has a ranula, which is mostly seen in young children and adolescents. A presentation such as this is unusual and you should be suspicious of other pathology. The marked atypia would suggest a small squamous cell carcinoma (SCC) obstructing the submandibular duct. The patient should be imaged, ideally by MR.

11. C. Lymphocyte. A patient with rheumatoid arthritis and a slowly enlarging parotid mass is likely to be suffering from Sjögren's syndrome. A discrete mass would be due to a MALT lymphoma, differentiating it from a diffuse swelling of the gland. This type of lymphoma is derived from B-lymphocytes.

12. C. The lesion originates from the parotid gland. Serous and myoepithelial cells are found in normal parotid tissue, but keratin deposition is a histological characteristic of SCC. Secondary metastatic deposits are the most common intraparotid pathology, but imaging would suggest this may be a primary lesion. Facial nerve involvement in primary salivary gland lesions is found in between 20 and 30% of cases but much more likely in primary SCC.

13. B. Extracorporeal lithotripsy. This patient has a stone in the middle third of the submandibular duct. The principal factor driving the presence of extracorporeal lithotripsy is its safety profile. A rough cut-off is that it can be used for stones up to 7 mm in diameter. The obvious limitations are its availability and the treatment duration, with successful cases needing multiple visits of up to an hour in length.

14. E. A neurilemoma should be suspected. This lesion likely represents a tumour in the pre-styloid component of the parapharyngeal space (PPS). The carotid space is the post-styloid PPS. Tumors of the PPS usually have to grow to at least 2.5–3 cm before they are detected. The primary radiological differential diagnosis for a tumor originating in the pre-styloid PPS is a pleomorphic adenoma (arising from the deep lobe of the parotid) or a neurilemoma (arising from the lingual nerve, inferior alveolar nerve, or auriculotemporal nerve). Concern of seeding from fine needle aspiration biopsy is unwarranted, but CT guidance is often required.

15. B. Nerve sparing surgery. Multinodular recurrence implies that at the primary surgery the wound bed was contaminated with tumour cells and that subsequent surgical resection alone cannot reliably eradicated residual disease. Should treatment be indicated then it should at least involve radiotherapy. Even in multinodular recurrence, disease progression can be so protracted that surveillance alone is a possible option, but it is the least preferable.

References

Armstrong JG, Harrison LB, Spiro RH, et al (1990). Malignant tumours of major salivary gland origin. A matched pair analysis of the role of combined surgery and postoperative radiotherapy. *Archives of Otorhinolaryngology-Head & Neck Surgery* **116**(3):290–293.

Combes J, Karavidas K, McGurk M (2009). Intraoral removal of proximal submandibular stones—an alternative to sialadenectomy? *British Journal of Oral and Maxillofacial Surgery* **38**(8):813–816.

Piedbois, Bataini J, Colin P, et al (1989). Conventional megavoltage radiotherapy in the management of malignant epithelial tumours of the parotid gland. *Radiotherapy & Oncology* **16**(3):203–209.

Terhaard CHJ, Lubsen H, Rasch CRN, et al (2005). The role of radiotherapy in the treatment of malignant salivary gland tumours. *International Journal of Radiation Oncology, Biology, Physics* **61**(1):103–111.

1. **A 76-year-old man with severe chronic obstructive pulmonary disease and schizophrenia is experiencing recurrent temporomandibular joint (TMJ) dislocation bilaterally, resulting in multiple hospital attendances per week. He is taking risperidone and quetiapine. What is the best management?**
   A. Autologous blood injection
   B. Prolotherapy with hypertonic dextrose
   C. Eminectomy
   D. Dautrey procedure
   E. A period of intermaxillary fixation (IMF)

2. **A 43-year-old woman with episodic pain and locking of her right TMJ has failed conservative management. Arthroscopy reveals a well-preserved joint space with early fibrillation. A large tear in the meniscus with exposure of the condylar head is seen and intra-articular steroid is placed at the time of the arthroscopy. Whilst there is transient symptomatic improvement, at 10 weeks she has returned to her baseline pain level of 7/10 on a visual analogue scale (VAS), with mouth opening of 33 mm. What is the next appropriate management step?**
   A. Repeat arthroscopy
   B. Intra-articular steroid injection in the outpatients clinic
   C. Intramuscular botulinum toxin injections to the ipsilateral lateral pterygoid muscle
   D. Meniscectomy
   E. Total alloplastic joint replacement

3. **A 36-year-old man with Wilkes III internal joint derangement of the left TMJ with limited mouth opening has a magnetic resonance imaging (MRI) scan that demonstrates anterior disc displacement. He undergoes an arthroscopy. What is the likelihood of improvement in mouth opening?**
   A. Less than 20%
   B. 20–40%
   C. 40–60%
   D. 60–80%
   E. Greater than 80%

4. **Which of the following steps is not a part of the Kaban protocol for the management of TMJ ankylosis in children?**
    A. Aggressive excision of the fibrous and/or bony mass
    B. Ipsilateral coronoidectomy
    C. Contralateral coronoidectomy
    D. Early mobilization
    E. Antibiotic-impregnated methacrylate spacer

5. **A patient with recurrent dislocation secondary to Ehlers–Danlos syndrome undergoes botulinum toxin injection to one of the muscles of mastication. Which muscle is targeted?**
    A. Masseter
    B. Temporalis
    C. Medial pterygoid
    D. Superior head of lateral pterygoid
    E. Inferior head of lateral pterygoid

6. **MRI of a patient with Wilkes III internal joint derangement symptoms shows a joint effusion. Which sequence would demonstrate this finding most conclusively?**
    A. T1-weighted
    B. T2-weighted
    C. Proton density weighted
    D. Short tau inversion recovery (STIR) sequence
    E. Fat sat pulsed MRI

7. **An orthopantomogram (OPG) shows advanced degenerative changes of the left TMJ suggestive of end-stage osteoarthritis, demonstrative pronounced flattening with osteophyte formation, and subcondylar sclerosis with significant loss of joint space. The patient complains of trismus and constant pain, rated as 8/10 in severity, well localized to the joint and aggravated by activities such as yawning and eating. Mouth opening is measured at 26 mm inter-incisal distance. What is the next best imaging modality choice?**
    A. Cone beam computed tomography (CBCT)
    B. Multidetector computed tomography (MDCT)
    C. Ultrasound (US)
    D. MRI
    E. Arthrogram

8. **A 43-year-old woman undergoes botulinum toxin injections for myofascial pain in her masseters bilaterally. A few days later she telephones to say that her smile is now asymmetrical. Which muscle is most likely to be affected?**

    A. Risorius
    B. Zygomaticus major
    C. Zygomaticus minor
    D. Orbicularis oris
    E. Depressor anguli oris

9. **A patient attends for intramuscular injection of botulinum toxin to the right masseter for hypertrophy. The standard practice of the clinician is to administer 30 units of Botox® to a masseter muscle. On the day, the pharmacy states that they only have Dysport® in stock. What is the corresponding dose?**

    A. 30 units
    B. 60 units
    C. 100 units
    D. 200 units
    E. 300 units

10. **A 74-year-old woman attends with a 1-year history of a swelling in front of the right ear. An MRI scan is shown in Figure 7.1. Clinical examination reveals a full range of movement of her TMJ, with mouth opening of 45 mm and pain scores of 2/10. An open biopsy of the joint (arthrotomy) yields multiple opalescent loose bodies, which are curetted away with ease. A well-preserved joint with no inflammation is visualized in the upper joint space. The reporting histopathologist advises that the differential diagnosis includes low-grade chondrosarcoma and 'atypical' synovial chondromatosis. What is the most appropriate course of action?**

    A. Serial clinical and radiographic review
    B. Radiotherapy
    C. Synovectomy
    D. Total alloplastic joint replacement
    E. Chemotherapy

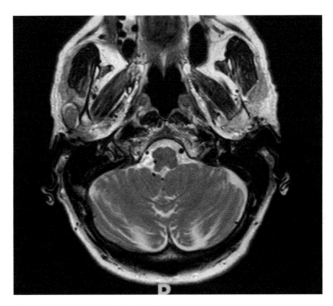

Figure 7.1 MRI of the temporomandibular joint.

11. **A 64-year-old man is due to undergo a total alloplastic joint replacement of the left TMJ with a custom TMJ Concepts device. He demonstrates a positive response to nickel on patch testing. What must you tell him in light of this?**
    A. He should proceed with a standard TMJ Concepts prosthesis
    B. Due to his allergy he is unable to have a prosthetic joint replacement
    C. He will require a device to be provided by an alternative manufacturer
    D. He will require an alternative fossa component from TMJ Concepts which has reduced stability on in vitro testing
    E. He will require an alternative ramus component from TMJ Concepts which demonstrates adverse wear characteristics.

12. **A 26-year-old man presents 4 months following blunt force trauma to the left side of his face (Figure 7.2). He complains of difficulty opening the mouth or eating anything hard, and ongoing pain around the left pre-auricular region, which he rates as 7/10 in severity on a VAS. He has been using ibuprofen 5% gel for the pain and some exercises that his general dental practitioner has given him. What is the next step in management?**
    A. Continued trial of conservative management
    B. Arthrocentesis
    C. Arthroscopy
    D. Open arthroplasty +/− meniscectomy
    E. Total prosthetic replacement of the left TMJ

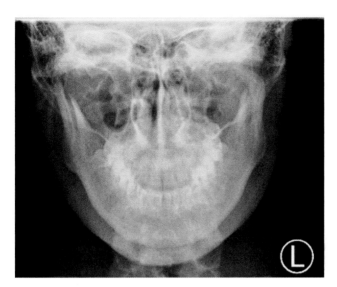

Figure 7.2 Plain radiograph of the face following trauma.

13. **Which of the following options of interposition arthroplasty materials are likely to be best suited to suppress heterotopic bone formation?**
    A. Silastic™
    B. Polymethyl methacrylate (PMMA) impregnated with antibiotics
    C. Temporalis muscle flap
    D. Autologous dermis-fat graft
    E. Homologous cartilage

14. **A patient is scheduled for an alloplastic total joint replacement (TJR) of the left TMJ, having previously undergone replacement of the contralateral joint many years prior. Three-dimensional (3D) reconstruction of the computed tomography (CT) scan data is shown in Figure 7.3. Which manufacturer is likely to have produced the preceding TJR?**
    A. TMJ Concepts
    B. Zimmer Biomet
    C. Engimplan
    D. Christensen
    E. OrthoTiN

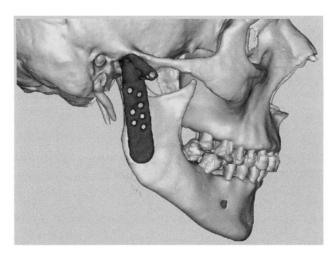

Figure 7.3 Three-dimensional planning for total joint replacement.

15. Which of the following is true of metal hypersensitivity to components of a total TMJ replacement?

A. If present, patient should be given an all-titanium prosthesis
B. It will be detected by skin patch testing
C. It may be detected by in vivo skin lymphocyte transformation test
D. It presents as recurrent swelling and infection
E. It is most commonly due to copper, chromium, or cobalt

1. B. Prolotherapy with hypertonic dextrose. Elledge and Speculand (2018) deal with non-surgical management of recurrent dislocation. Generally, simpler measures should be tried first, particularly in elderly patients with multiple co-morbidities. Autologous blood is a good option but can lead to marked fibrosis and trismus. Prolotherapy can be done in the outpatients setting using intra-articular and peri-articular injections of a safe non-sclerosant material such as 20% or 50% dextrose.

2. D. Meniscectomy. With a large tear in the meniscus and exposure of the condylar head, repeat arthroscopy is unlikely to be successful (although arthroscopically assisted repair of the disc might be attempted). Realistically with such identifiable pathology, open arthroplasty and likely meniscectomy with a free fat graft would be a good next step in management for the relatively well-preserved joint save for an unsalvageable meniscus.

3. E. Greater than 80%. Ahmed et al (2012) published outcomes from a large cohort of patients and demonstrated 82% improvement in mouth opening for this subgroup, a finding echoed elsewhere in the literature.

4. E. Antibiotic-impregnated methacrylate spacer. Methacrylate spacers are used in infected joints requiring removal and adult gap arthroplasties, but are not featured in the Kaban protocol which features all the other answers but stresses in particular the importance of aggressive early mobilization of the joint and physiotherapy.

5. E. Inferior head of lateral pterygoid. There are a number of conservative treatment strategies for recurrent TMJ dislocation including prolotherapy, sclerosant injection, autologous blood injection, and botulinum toxin. The inferior head of the lateral pterygoid is a strong contributor to mandibular protrusion. Ideally this is targeted with electromyography (EMG) guidance to avoid complications such as dysphagia.

6. B. T2-weighted. T2-weighted MRI shows effusions particularly well. Fat suppression techniques such as STIR are good for showing marrow oedema of the condyle and accentuating fluid.

7. B. Multidetector helical computed tomogram (MDCT). CT would be the imaging modality of choice for examining the hard tissue structures of established arthritis. Whilst CBCT would yield diagnostic information with limited radiation exposure, with the parameters described the patient is arguably a candidate for a total joint replacement. CT scan would enable fabrication of a custom total joint replacement by the two manufacturers approved for use in the UK: TMJ Concepts and Zimmer Biomet.

8. B. Zygomaticus major. Facial asymmetry most commonly results from injections being sited too high up and anterior on the masseter muscle. This tends to affect the zygomaticus major muscle most frequently.

9. C. 100 units. Conversion rates vary throughout the literature for Botox® and Dysport® from 6:1 to 1:1, although generally a conversion rate of 3:1 (Dysport® to Botox®) is regarded as approaching the most accurate figure. The author's practice currently is to use around 30–50 units of Botox® in a masseter and 25–30 units in a temporalis muscle.

10. A. Serial clinical and radiographic review. Recommended treatment options for synovial chondromatosis have included removal of the foreign bodies by either arthroscopy or open arthrotomy, synovectomy, condylectomy, discectomy, and reconstruction with costochondral graft with pedicled deep temporal fascial fat flap. The evidence base is restricted to case reports and case series, although generally in well-preserved joints (as is the case here), treatment is conservative and restricted to removal of loose bodies and partial synovectomy in the presence of marked inflammation. Malignant transformation is exceptionally rare, with only three cases described in the English literature.

11. E. He will require an alternative ramus component from TMJ Concepts which demonstrates adverse wear characteristics. The all-titanium version of the bespoke prosthesis from TMJ Concepts has not been Food and Drug Administration (FDA) approved in the United States and patients must sign an additional disclaimer regarding potential adverse wear and poorer evidence regarding longevity of the devices.

12. E. Total prosthetic replacement of the left TMJ. This man has a fracture-dislocation of the left condyle, which has been left untreated, resulting in a malunion, with the condylar head displaced medially out of the glenoid fossa. Given the diagnosis and the parameters of his pain score and restriction of opening, the only available option is a joint replacement if conservative management has failed to address his symptoms. Indications for this are set out in a position paper by Andrew Sidebottom (2008) on behalf of the British Association of TMJ Surgeons (BATS).

13. D. Autologous dermis-fat graft. Whilst the debate surrounding the 'ideal' interpositional material in TMJ gap arthroplasty is far from settled, there is a body of evidence to suggest that re-ankylosis and heterotopic bone formation is suppressed by autologous fat grafting. This is summarized nicely in a systematic review by van Bogaert et al. (2018).

14. D. Christensen. There are a broad range of devices available on the market and these are covered by Elledge et al. (2019). TMJ surgeons in the UK currently use ether TMJ Concepts or Zimmer Biomet devices, with robust long-term data now available for both systems.

15. A. If present, patient should be given an all-titanium prosthesis. Despite their biocompatibility with most patients, some of the metals that provide strength to the joint replacements are also considered common allergens, including nickel, chromium, and cobalt. Symptoms include recurrent swelling in the absence of infection or refractory neuropathic-like pain. The two most commonly used tests are the in vivo skin patch test and in vitro lymphocyte transformation test. However, although widely performed, routine testing is not supported by the literature.

References

Ahmed N, Sidebottom A, O'Connor M, Kerr HL (2012). Prospective outcome assessment of the therapeutic benefits of arthroscopy and arthrocentesis of the temporomandibular joint. *British Journal of Oral and Maxillofacial Surgery* **50**(8):745–748.

Elledge ROC, Speculand B (2018). Conservative management options for dislocation of the temporomandibular joint. In: Matthews NS (ed.) *Dislocation of the Temporomandibular Joint*, 63–70. Cham: Springer.

Elledge R, Mercuri LG, Attard A, et al (2019). Review of emerging temporomandibular joint total joint replacement systems. *British Journal of Oral and Maxillofacial Surgery* **57**(8):722–728.

Sidebottom A (2008). Guidelines for the replacement of temporomandibular joints in the United Kingdom. *British Journal of Oral and Maxillofacial Surgery* **46**(2):146–147.

van Bogaert W, de Meurechy N, Mommaerts MY (2018). Autologous far grafting in total temporomandibular joint replacement surgery. *Annals of Maxillofacial Surgery* **8**(2):299–302.

1. Following a dental extraction, a 78-year-old man with a previous history of multiple myeloma develops exposed bone with intermittent purulent discharge in the right hemimandible. Radiographs demonstrate regions of osteosclerosis of the alveolar bone with obscuring of the periodontal ligament of adjacent teeth. What is the recommended management?

    A. Sequestrectomy
    B. Pentoxifylline, tocopherol, and clodronate (PENTOCLO) combination therapy
    C. Hyperbaric oxygen therapy
    D. Chlorohexidine gluconate 0.12% mouthwash
    E. Chlorohexidine gluconate 0.12% mouthwash and oral doxycycline

2. A unilocular lesion around the crown of an unerupted lower left third molar is enucleated in a 25-year-old woman with an otherwise sound dentition. Histology demonstrates a unicystic ameloblastoma with nodular proliferation into the lumen of the lesion but no infiltration of tumour cells into the connective tissue wall. What is the next most appropriate management?

    A. Serial clinical and radiographic review
    B. Re-enucleation with peripheral ostectomy
    C. Re-enucleation with Carnoy's solution
    D. Rim resection of the mandible
    E. Segmental resection of the mandible ensuring 1 cm clearance

3. A cyst related to the apical portion of a carious tooth is enucleated from the right maxilla. Whilst presumed to be a radicular cyst, histopathology demonstrates findings in keeping with a keratocyst. A supplemental report suggests that this is an orthokeratinized variant. What is the next most appropriate step in management?

    A. Serial clinical and radiographic review
    B. Repeat curettage of the area and peripheral ostectomy
    C. Repeat curettage and Carnoy's solution
    D. Repeat curettage and cryotherapy
    E. Segmental resection (partial maxillectomy)

4. **A 19-year-old with a biopsy-confirmed keratocyst of the mandible is weighing up treatment options, making the decision in conjunction with yourself balancing treatment aggressiveness with recurrence rate. Which of the following treatment modalities would yield the lowest recurrence rate?**

A. Marsupialization
B. Decompression and enucleation
C. Enucleation alone
D. Enucleation with peripheral ostectomy
E. Enucleation with Carnoy's solution

5. **A 37-year-old man presents with recurrent episodes of trismus and swelling of the right mandible over a period of 4 years with no history of trauma or infection. Plain radiographs demonstrate unilateral diffuse sclerosis affecting the ipsilateral hemimandible. A biopsy shows no organisms on microscopy or culture, but reveals devitalized bony fragments with fibro-collagenous tissue and lymphocyte infiltration. Which of the following would not be a recognized treatment?**

A. Hyperbaric oxygen
B. Surgical debridement
C. Subcutaneous calcitonin
D. Denosumab
E. Bevacizumab

6. **A 23-year-old man attends with pain in the left hemimandible and a radiograph reveals appearances as shown in Figure 8.1. What would be your recommended management?**

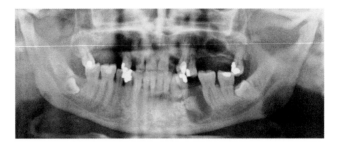

Figure 8.1 OPG radiograph demonstrating bone abnormality.

A. Decompression with grommet insertion
B. Enucleation
C. Enucleation with Carnoy's solution
D. Enucleation with peripheral ostectomy
E. Segmental resection

7. **A 34-year-old woman presents with a swelling of the right maxilla. Plain film radiographs reveal a well-defined radiolucency, and histology from curettage of the lesion demonstrates vascular connective tissue with focally aggregate multinucleated giant cells. Her parathyroid hormone level is found to be significantly raised. What is the next investigation of choice?**
    A. Repeat plain film radiographs
    B. Computed tomography (CT) scan
    C. Magnetic resonance imaging (MRI) scan
    D. Technetium-99m (99mTc) sestamibi scan
    E. Positron emission tomography (PET) scan

8. **The patient shown in Figure 8.2 is currently being treated with subcutaneous denosumab. Her tooth-borne partial denture is now too painful to wear, but the pain resolves when removed. On gentle probing of the lump you can feel uneven bone below. Which of the following is true?**

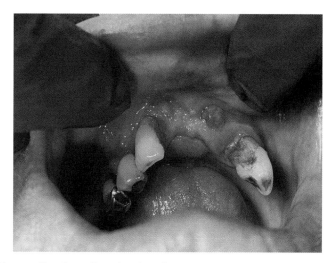

Figure 8.2 Abnormality of maxillary alveolar ridge.

    A. The denosumab dose should be changed to oral
    B. This event should be reported to the Medicines Control Agency
    C. The fit surface of the denture should be modified and immediately replaced
    D. Consideration of bone saucerization is recommended at this stage
    E. Pamidronate is an alternative treatment with similar risks

9. The patient with the image shown in Figure 8.3 presents with pus
    draining from a chronic cutaneous fistula. He was hit in the face
    3 months previously but did not seek treatment. Which of the following
    is correct about the causative organisms?

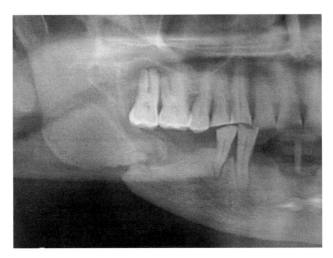

Figure 8.3 OPG radiograph of a patient with previous facial trauma.

   A. They are likely due to a virulent organism
   B. They are similar to that found in long bone fractures
   C. They are predominantly a single organism, requiring targeted antibiotic therapy
   D. They are predominantly opportunistic and aerobic
   E. They are most commonly *Staphylococcus aureus*

10. During incisional biopsy, the lesion shown in Figure 8.4 was found to
    be easily dissectable from bone. Enucleation was performed which
    was believed to be complete. Histology demonstrated intraluminal
    plexiform proliferation of the epithelium. Which is the most appropriate
    management?
   A. Observation
   B. Repeat enucleation followed by curettage
   C. Curretage alone
   D. Cryotherapy to the cystic cavity
   E. Resection with 1-cm margin

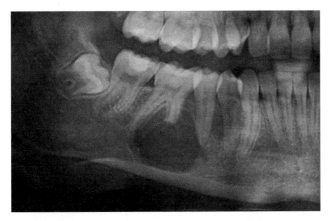

Figure 8.4 Part of an OPG radiograph showing mandibular radiolucency.

11. **A 60-year-old man is sent in by his dentist with the following appearance on his radiograph (Figure 8.5). He is experiencing pain and altered lip sensation but is otherwise well. Biopsy demonstrates large numbers of abnormal plasma cells. What is the most important next step in management?**

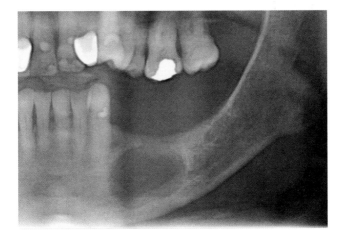

Figure 8.5 Part of an OPG radiograph demonstrating radiolucency.

    A. CT scan of facial bones to identify other deposits
    B. Whole body MRI
    C. Serology to detect hypocalcaemia
    D. Curettage of mandibular lesion
    E. Whole body CT scan

12. Which of the following treatment options for the patient shown in Figure 8.6 has the lowest incidence for subsequent recurrence and side effects?

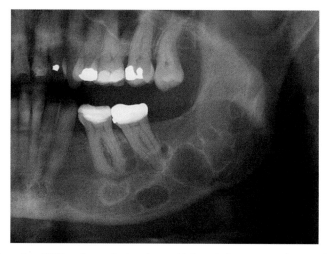

Figure 8.6 Part of an OPG radiograph showing multiple radiolucencies in the mandible.

    A. Peripheral ostectomy after curettage
    B. En bloc resection
    C. Enucleation followed by cryotherapy
    D. Decompression followed by enucleation
    E. Topical application of 5-FU after enucleation

13. The biopsy enucleation of a solid lump in the anterior mandible comes back as eosinophillic granuloma. What is the correct treatment?
    A. Chemotherapy
    B. Surveillance
    C. Resection with a 5-mm margin
    D. Resection with a 10-mm margin
    E. Radiotherapy

14. A 37-year-old patient presents with a pathological mandibular fracture associated with a 3-cm radiolucency. The histology is shown in Figure 8.7 and includes giant cells. Which of the following is *not* a differential diagnosis?
    A. Brown tumour
    B. Primary hyperparathyroidism
    C. Aneurysmal bone cyst
    D. Osteosarcoma
    E. Odontogenic keratocyst

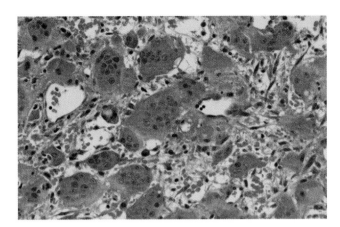

Figure 8.7 Histology of patient on presentation.

15. A 15-year-old girl presents with an unerupted impacted right maxillary canine. Radiographs demonstrate an 11-mm unilocular radiolucency encompassing the crown. Which one of the following is the most likely diagnosis?

A. Dentigerous cyst

B. Unicystic ameloblastoma

C. Lateral periodontal cyst

D. Adenomatoid odontogenic tumour

E. Radicular cyst

1. E. Chlorohexidine gluconate 0.12% mouthwash and oral doxycycline. As someone with previous myeloma, the presumption here is that it is medication-related osteonecrosis of the jaw (MRONJ) secondary to bisphosphonates. He is Ruggiero stage II, and as such, recommendations from the 2014 position paper by Ruggiero and colleagues on behalf of the American Association of Oral and Maxillofacial Surgeons (AAOMS) would be for a chlorohexidine mouth rinse and oral antimicrobials.

2. A. Serial clinical and radiographic review. Unicystic ameloblastomas which show no intramural invasion (i.e. simple and intraluminal subtypes of the unicystic variant) can be safely managed by enucleation alone with ongoing follow-up. Indeed, the diagnosis is often made retrospectively. A good review is provided by Parmar et al. (2016).

3. A. Serial clinical and radiographic review. The orthokeratinized variant of keratocysts is presumed by some to be a distinct pathological entity from the conventional parakeratinized keratocyst. It has a much lower recurrence rate, and enucleation would be an acceptable treatment option given the supplemental report.

4. E. Enucleation with Carnoy's solution. There is a balance to be struck in terms of aggressiveness versus acceptable recurrence rates in treating keratocysts. Generally, most authorities would agree that more conservative options should be tried first, with options such as segmental resection held in reserve. Adjuncts such as peripheral ostectomy and Carnoy's reduce recurrence rates, the latter more effectively, as highlighted in a systematic review of 6,427 cases by Chrcanovic and Gomez (2017).

5. E. Bevacizumab. The clinical picture, histology, and radiographs, particularly the absence of an infective focus, point towards diffuse sclerosing osteomyelitis (DSO). There is little in the way of consensus regarding management, but case reports and series suggest all the possibilities A–D, but not bevacizumab, which is an antivascular endothelial growth factor (VEGF-A) monoclonal antibody. A comprehensive review has recently been published by van de Meent et al. (2020).

6. B. Enucleation. The appearances are in keeping with a compound odontome with discrete radio-opaque 'denticles' demonstrated within a wider radiolucent lesion. Treatment is enucleation of the lesion, which is regarded as curative, with low recurrence rates reported.

7. D. Technetium-99m (99mTc) sestamibi scan. The differentiation between a central giant cell granuloma and brown tumour of hyperparathyroidism is impossible to make histologically. Once the latter is demonstrated, a 99mTc sestamibi scan is advisable to attempt to localize a parathyroid adenoma.

8. C. The fit surface of the denture should be modified and immediately replaced.
This patient has stage 1 MRONJ. Clinical practice guidelines published by Yarom et al. (2019) state that both pamidronate and denosumab can be used for solid organ tumours, but the former has a far higher risk of developing MRONJ (3.2–5.03% versus 0.7–6.9%). The fit surface of a tooth-borne denture can be adjusted without having to wait for 3 months. Suspected adverse drug reactions should be reported to the Medicines and Healthcare products Regulatory Agency (MHRA).

9. B. They are similar to that found in long bone fractures. This patient likely has a non- union and chronic osteomyelitis following previous mandible fracture. In non- traumatic cases the organisms resemble those found in odontogenic infections (i.e. a polymicrobial, opportunistic infection, caused primarily by a mixture of alpha haemolytic streptococci and anaerobic bacteria from the oral cavity). However, following trauma, osteomyelitis of the mandible it is more likely due to *Staphylococcus epidermis* (unlike osteomyelitis of the long bones, which are usually caused by *Staphylococcus aureus*).

10. A. Observation. This patient has a unicystic ameloblastoma, the histology of which would support Grade 2 of Ackermann's classification. Based upon an incisional biopsy, the generally accepted treatment is enucleation and curettage, with frequent follow-up examinations. However, as this patient has already had enucleation alone, there is limited evidence to support repeat surgery with curettage or cryotherapy.

11. B. Whole body MRI. This patient likely has multiple myeloma and a CT scan of the facial bones may show other deposits, although this is relatively unlikely. More importantly, the patient requires a skeletal survey, serology testing, and a bone marrow biopsy. Early disease limited to marrow may go undetected at CT scan but is usually seen on MRI, with whole body MRI recommended to determine the extent of disease. Myeloma lesions appear as low signal intensity lesions on T1-weighted MRI and hyperintense on T2-weighted MRI.

12. D. Decompression followed by enucleation. This lesion most likely represents an odontogenic keratocyst. All of these treatments are effective. A systematic review by Sharif et al (2015) found no high-quality evidence to suggest one treatment over another. Unilocular and small multilocular lesions are generally treated more conservatively through enucleation and curettage. Although decompression followed by enucleation likely has lower recurrence, the risk of nerve damage between treatments appears similar.

13. C. Resection with a 5-mm margin. Eosinophilic granuloma, formerly known as histiocytosis X, is now classed as a neoplastic process, mostly affecting boys under the age of 10. Treatment of localized accessible lesions is with aggressive curettage or resection with 5-mm margins where possible. Involved mobile teeth should be removed, although vitality is often preserved. Inaccessible lesions can be treated with radiotherapy. Disseminated disease is often lethal and treatment is with chemotherapy. Intralesional steroid injections produce regression of localized lesions. Clinical and radiological monitoring is needed.

14. E. Odontogenic keratocyst. You will be unlikely to be asked much histology, with the exception of obvious slides such as immunofluorescence in bullous lesions, or in this slide which shows giant cells. Giant cell (Brown) tumours, giant cell granulomas, aneurysmal bone cysts, and some osteosarcomas show similar macroscopic and microscopic features.

15.   A. Dentigerous cyst.   A pericoronal radiolucency associated with an impacted canine is most likely to represent a dentigerous cyst. An adenomatoid odontogenic tumour would be expected to envelop both the crown and roots.

References

Chrcanovic BR, Gomez RS (2017). Recurrence probability for keratocystic odontogenic tumours: an analysis of 6,427 cases. *Journal of Cranio-Maxillofacial Surgery* **45**:244–251.

Parmar S, Al-Qamachi L, Aga H (2016). Ameloblastomas of the mandible and maxilla. *Current Opinion in Otolaryngology & Head and Neck Surgery* **24**:148–154.

Ruggiero SL, Dodson TB, Fantasia J, et al (2014). American Association of Oral and Maxillofacial Surgeons position paper on medication-related osteonecrosis of the jaw—2014 update. *Journal of Oral and Maxillofacial Surgery* **72**:1938–1956.

Sharif FNJ, Oliver R, Sweet C, Sharif MO (2015). Interventions for the treatment of keratocystic odontogenic tumours. *Cochrane Database of Systematic Reviews* **11**:CD008464.

van de Meent MM, Pichardo SEC, Appelman-Dijkstra NM, van Merkesteyn JPR (2020). Outcome of different treatments for chronic diffuse sclerosing osteomyelitis of the mandible: a systematic review of published papers. *British Journal of Oral and Maxillofacial Surgery* **58**(4):385–395.

Yarom N, Shapiro CL, Peterson DE, et al (2019). Medication-related osteonecrosis of the jaw (MRONJ): MASCC/ISOO/ASCO clinical practice guideline. *Journal of Clinical Oncology* **37**(25):2270–2290.

1. **A 56-year-old woman presents with a painful atrophic area on the right buccal mucosa. Biopsy confirms lichenoid interface mucositis with no evidence of dysplasia. She has no adjacent restorations and treatment with soluble prednisolone 5 mg in 15 ml water as a mouthwash proves ineffective. What is the next logical step in management?**
   A. Systemic azathioprine
   B. Systemic prednisolone
   C. Topical ciclosporin 100 mg/ml as mouthwash twice daily
   D. Clobetasol propionate 0.05% ointment
   E. Topical tacrolimus (Protopic 0.03%)

2. **A 35-year-old woman complains of multiple sore, erosive areas affecting her buccal mucosa bilaterally and hard palate. Nikolsky's sign is positive on examination. What is the most sensitive diagnostic test?**
   A. Indirect immunofluorescence testing
   B. Haematoxylin and eosin staining of affected mucosa
   C. Haematoxylin and eosin staining of unaffected mucosa
   D. Direct immunofluorescence staining of affected mucosa
   E. Direct immunofluorescence staining of unaffected mucosa

3. **A 68-year-old woman presents with gradually increasing swelling and pain of the tongue. Examination reveals a sharply demarcated area of colour change to the distal third of the tongue with obvious ischaemia. A vasculitis screen, electrocardiogram (ECG), and computed tomography (CT) angiogram are unremarkable, but erythrocyte sedimentation rate (ESR) is raised at 55 mm/hour. What is the next step in management?**
   A. Empirical antibiotic treatment
   B. Intravenous unfractionated heparin
   C. Thrombolysis
   D. High-dose steroids
   E. Therapeutic low molecular weight heparin (LMWH)

4. A 64-year-old woman develops widespread oral bullae and ulceration and sore eyes after a course of vancomycin. In addition, she develops an annular rash on her trunk and limbs, demonstrating a 'string of pearls' sign, appearing as blisters around wheal-like red patches. What is the initial treatment likely to be?

    A. Dapsone
    B. Mycophenolate mofetil
    C. Colchicine
    D. Ciclosporin
    E. Doxycycline

5. A 7-year-old girl attends with multiple sessile papules involving the upper labial mucosa and buccal mucosa ranging from 2 to 10 mm in diameter. An excisional biopsy of one of the lesions reveals squamous epithelium with verrucous proliferation, marked papillomatosis, perinuclear cellular vacuolization (koilocytosis), and isolated mitosoid cells. Polymerase chain reaction (PCR) testing demonstrates human papillomavirus (HPV) subtype 32 deoxyribonucleic acid (DNA). What is the next step in management?

    A. No further management
    B. Safeguarding referral
    C. Cryotherapy
    D. Carbon dioxide laser ablation
    E. Topical treatment with interferon-alpha and retinoic acid

6. A 50-year-old woman presents with a solitary slow-growing lesion on the hard palate, which is sessile and firm on examination with normal overlying mucosa. The lesion is excised and submitted for histopathology, which demonstrates a marginal excision with 'plywood-like' clefts between collagen bundles and fibroblasts exhibiting spindle-shaped nuclei arranged in a storiform ('cartwheel') pattern. Staining is positive for CD34 with a 'fingerprint-like' pattern. What further management is required?

    A. No further management
    B. Staging CT scan of the neck and thorax
    C. Wider excision with fenestration of the hard palate
    D. Adjuvant radiotherapy
    E. Referral for genetic counselling

7. **A 10-year-old boy presents with unilateral cervical lymphadenopathy which appeared in the days following a scratch from his grandmother's pet. A core biopsy demonstrates follicular hyperplasia and non-specific granulomatous inflammation. PCR identifies DNA of a specific organism that confirms the suspected diagnosis. Which organism?**
    A. Mycobacterium tuberculosis
    B. Actinomyces israelii
    C. Borrelia burgdorferi
    D. Bartonella henselae
    E. Treponema pallidum

8. **A 35-year-old man suffers recurrent attacks of severe unilateral headaches around the eye and temple, which he describes as 'stabbing'. The headaches have happened two to three times each day for the past week, each time lasting for around 60 minutes. His wife has noticed some ipsilateral ptosis and tearing during the attacks. What would be a recommended first-line preventive agent?**
    A. Lamotrigine
    B. Carbamazepine
    C. Verapamil
    D. Sumatriptan
    E. Indomethacin

9. **Pentoxifylline may be used in combination with tocopherol (vitamin E) in the treatment of osteoradionecrosis (ORN). Which of the following statements is *not* true concerning pentoxifylline?**
    A. It is a methylated xanthine derivative
    B. It scavenges reactive oxygen species
    C. It is a phosphodiesterase inhibitor
    D. It inhibits tumour necrosis factor (TNF) alpha
    E. It increases erythrocyte flexibility

10. **Which of the following options does *not* refer to an eponymous staging system for the severity of ORN?**
    A. Marx
    B. Notani
    C. Ruggiero
    D. Epstein
    E. Lyons

11. A 29-year-old man attends with a bluish swelling above the left eyebrow measuring 11 mm in diameter present for the past few months. An excisional biopsy demonstrates areas of papillary endothelial hyperplasia and a diagnosis of a Masson's tumour is returned, with excision being marginal but complete. What is the next step in management?

A. No further management
B. Re-excision with 1-cm margin
C. Adjuvant radiotherapy
D. CT scan of the neck and thorax
E. Positron emission tomography (PET) scan

12. A 55-year-old woman presents with severe lancinating pain affecting her right cheek, manifesting as 'attacks' lasting for seconds at a time and precipitated by light touch and applying her make-up. Clinical examination and plain film radiographs exclude an odontogenic cause and she denies any autonomic symptoms. What would be the pharmacological therapy of choice?

A. Carbamazepine
B. Lamotrigine
C. Baclofen
D. Phenytoin
E. Amitriptyline

13. Biopsy of the lesion shown in Figure 9.1 demonstrates marked pleomorphic cells, frequent mitotic activity, and intercellular bridging. No keratin pearls are visible. Which of the following is the most likely diagnosis?

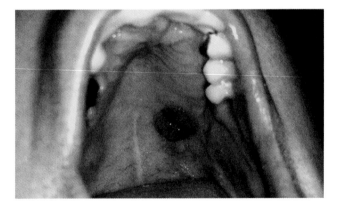

Figure 9.1 Lesion in the palate.

A. Adenocarcinoma
B. Poorly differentiated squamous cell carcinoma (SCC)
C. Adenoid cystic carcinoma
D. Well-differentiated SCC
E. Mucoepidermoid carcinoma

14. **Biopsy of this long-standing lesion on the right lateral tongue 6 months ago demonstrated a band-like lymphocytic infiltrate (Figure 9.2). The lesion has recently started swelling and repeat biopsy shows the presence of cells with an increased nuclear-to-cytoplasmic ratio now breaching the basement membrane. What is true of this process?**

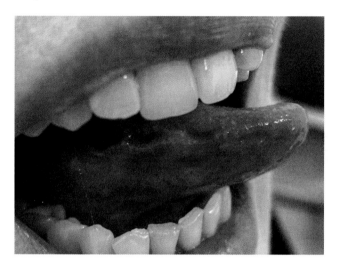

Figure 9.2 Inflamed tongue showing teeth indentation.

    A. The lifetime risk of this occurring in such a lesion is approximately 5%
    B. The original lesion most likely demonstrated plaque-like areas
    C. It more likely occurs in the floor of the mouth
    D. Hepatitis C virus infection increases the probability of it occurring
    E. Recurrence of the result pathology is more likely when no pre-existing lesion is present

15. **The patient shown in Figure 9.3 states that this discolouration on her lower lip has been present for 6 months. She was a long-term cigarette smoker but stopped when the lesions first appeared. She takes citalopram.**

    A. The patient should be reassured and reviewed in 6 months
    B. It is due to increased numbers of melanocytes
    C. Biopsy is required to confirm the diagnosis
    D. Serology should be taken for human immunodeficiency virus (HIV) positivity
    E. Advise changing the citalopram for another drug

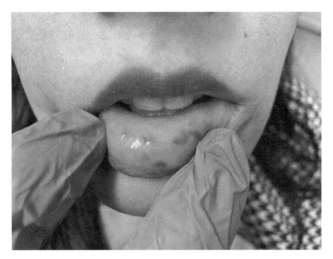

Figure 9.3 Pigmentation of the lower lip.

16. **The patient shown in Figure 9.4 returns following incisional biopsy of this tongue lesion. Histology demonstrates fibroepithelial hyperplasia with eosinophilic ulceration. Additional features associated with this presentation include which of the following?**

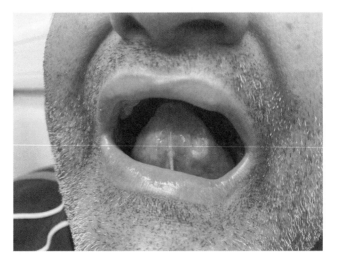

Figure 9.4 Ulceration under the tongue.

    A. Painless skin ulcers
    B. Vertigo
    C. Bright-red rectal bleeding
    D. Corneal perforation
    E. Shortness of breath

17. A patient presents with fever, headache, periorbital swelling, and diplopia. You suspect the cause is an infection most likely from:

A. Ethmoidal sinusitis

B. Dental abscess

C. Cranial valve abscess

D. Cardiac valve abscess

E. Nasal furuncle

18. Biopsy of the central part of the lesion shown in Figure 9.5 is likely to demonstrate what histological features?

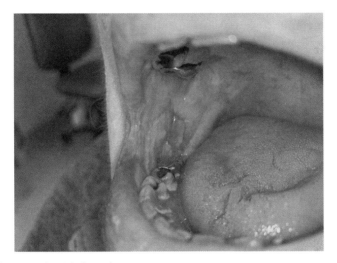

Figure 9.5 Lesion in the right buccal mucosa.

A. Hydropic degeneration of the basal cells

B. Scattered dyskeratotic keratinocytes

C. Neutrophils predominating over lymphocytes

D. A band-like lymphocytic infiltrate along the basement zone

E. Fibrosis and granuloma formation

19. You have been referred a patient following a failed extraction of a mandibular molar tooth. The patient is experiencing a unilateral paroxysmal throbbing headache affecting the whole side of their face, with disturbed vision. Which of the following is true?

A. Sensitivity to light would be expected

B. Treatment includes a carbonic anhydrase inhibitor

C. Caffeine should be avoided

D. Metoprolol would be more effective than carbamazepine

E. Ergotamine is a first line treatment

20. **A patient presents with a 2-cm oral ulcer in the palate. He was contacted by his last partner 6 months ago to say they had likely contracted an infection due to *Treponema pallidum*. Which of the following features is most diagnostic of this condition?**
    A. Non-response to intramuscular penicillin
    B. Recent serpingous oral ulceration
    C. Transmission of infection to a recent partner
    D. A treponemal test in conjunction with a non-treponemal test
    E. Dark-field microscopic examination to detect spirochetes

21. **A 25-year-old woman presents with a 3-month history of the isolated swelling shown in Figure 9.6. It does not bleed and is not changing in size. Management options include all the following except:**

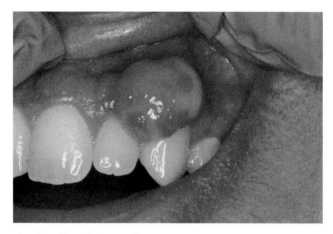

Figure 9.6 Localized swelling of the maxillary gingiva.

    A. Full blood count
    B. Subgingival debridement
    C. Laser excision
    D. Scalpel excision
    E. Pregnancy test

22. **You are asked to see the patient in Figure 9.7 on the high dependency unit. They have been struggling to eat due to pain inside the mouth for the last 4 days. They are receiving continuous positive airway pressure ventilation for pneumonia. They are currently on intravenous piperacillin with tazobactam. Which of the following is true?**
    A. Concurrent lesions on the torso are likely
    B. Intravenous acyclovir is indicated
    C. Oral acyclovir should be started
    D. The patient should be treated in a side room
    E. PCR testing is required to make a diagnosis

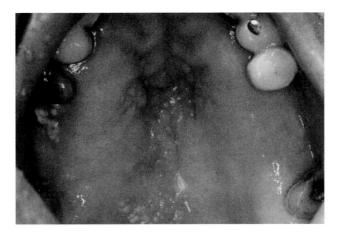

Figure 9.7 Appearance of the hard palate.

23. **Which of the following is _not_ a potentially malignant condition for SCC affecting the floor of the mouth?**
    A. Dyskeratosis congenita
    B. Syphilis
    C. Graft versus host disease
    D. Fanconi anaemia
    E. HIV

24. **This white patch on the tongue has increased in size over the last year (Figure 9.8). Biopsy demonstrates cellular atypia and loss of normal maturation and stratification present in over two-thirds of the epithelium. What does this represent?**
    A. Moderate dysplasia
    B. Atypical hyperplasia
    C. Squamous cell hyperplasia
    D. Carcinoma in situ
    E. Severe dysplasia

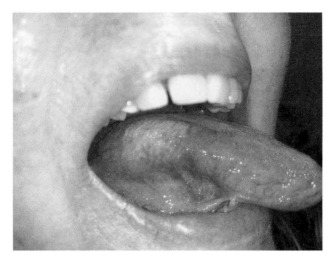

Figure 9.8 Leukoplakia on the right lateral border of the tongue.

25. A patient presents with this appearance on the attached gingivae (Figure 9.9). There are associated skin lesions. Autoantibodies to BP180 are identified. What is the diagnosis?

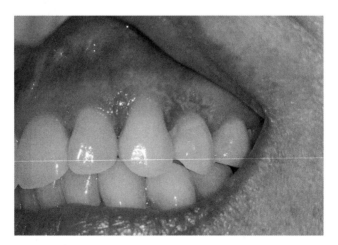

Figure 9.9 Appearance of the attached gingiva.

    A. Linear immunoglobulin A (IgA) disease
    B. Pemphigus
    C. Bullous pemphigoid
    D. Mucous membrane pemphigoid
    E. Cicatricial pemphigoid.

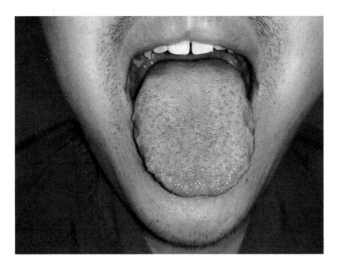

Figure 9.10 Appearance of the patient's tongue.

26. **This patient describes a 2-month history of a hot sensation affecting their tongue, lips, and palate (Figure 9.10). They are struggling to sleep. No pathology is found on examination. Which of the following treatments is *not* recommended?**

    A. Topical clonezapam
    B. Oral clonezapam
    C. Topical capsaicin
    D. Oral trazodone
    E. Oral nortriptyline

27. **The patient in Figure 9.11 presents with a worsening white patch on his tongue that has been present as long as he can remember. Examination of his nails demonstrates longitudinal ridging. Which of the following statements best represents this condition?**

    A. Full blood count will be normal
    B. Skin pigmentation is likely
    C. The rate of malignant transformation of this lesion is 5–10%.
    D. Bone marrow transplant will reduce the chance of death from associated malignancies
    E. The underlying pathology is telomere lengthening

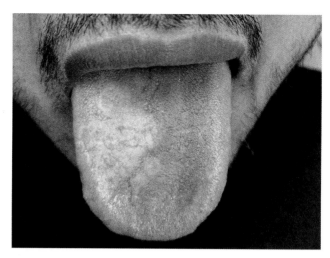

Figure 9.11 White appearance of the dorsum of the tongue.

28. **The 76-year-old patient shown in Figure 9.12 is 3 days following extraction of a lower right tooth and exploration of tissue spaces. She is a poorly controlled diabetic with stage 2 renal failure. The C-reactive protein (CRP) and white cell counts remain raised and the area of skin necrosis appears to be increasing in size. Which of the additional following parameters is of relevance?**

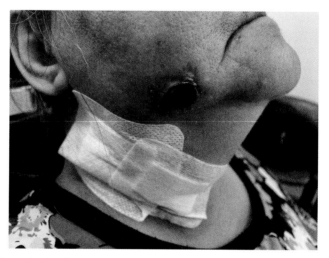

Figure 9.12 Right cheek inflammation and necrosis.

    A. Glucose
    B. Creatinine
    C. Haemoglobin
    D. Potassium
    E. Urea

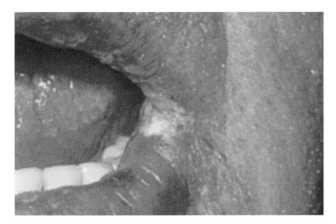

Figure 9.13 Mucosal changes at the angle of the mouth.

29. **Incisional biopsy of this lesion (Figure 9.13) that has been unresponsive to topical antimycotics demonstrates an acute inflammatory reaction, fungal hyphae, and severe dysplasia. What is the most appropriate next step?**
    A. Systemic antimycotics
    B. Photodynamic therapy
    C. Erbium:yttrium-aluminium-garnet (Er:YAG) laser
    D. Surgical vermilionectomy
    E. Systemic corticosteroids

30. **The patient shown in Figure 9.14 has been struggling to eat and his body mass index is 18. Nasogastric (NG) feeding with a standard polymeric feed is planned. Which of the following is true?**
    A. Pre-operative urea and electrolyte levels stratify patients at risk
    A. This patient should have a percutaneous endoscopic gastrostomy (PEG) inserted instead
    B. The patient should have regular albumin and vitamin D levels checked post-operatively
    C. The start of feeding should be deferred for at least 48 hours
    E. Post-operative hypophosphataemia or hypomagnesaemia should instigate slowing of NG feeding

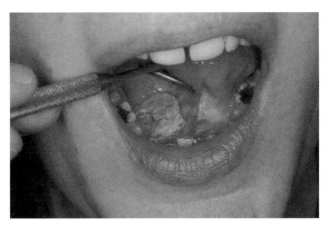

Figure 9.14 Appearance of lesion under the tongue.

1. D. Clobetasol propionate 0.05% ointment. British Society of Oral Medicine (BSOM) guidance recommends that with a focused area of lichen planus refractory to standard treatment, a topical potent steroid such as clobetasol propionate would be the next step in management before considering immunosuppressant agents and/or systemic steroids.

2. E. Direct immunofluorescence staining of unaffected mucosa. Nikolsky's sign being positive would imply pemphigus vulgaris rather than mucous membrane pemphigoid. The important consideration is that adjacent normal mucosa is sampled to enable detection of acantholysis as a result of antibodies directed against desmoglein-1 and desmoglein-3.

3. D. High-dose steroids. Distal tongue necrosis is an uncommon but recognized feature (and in some instances the presenting symptom) of giant cell or temporal arteritis. The key is the index of suspicion and absence of alternative explanations, along with the patient being the right demographic. Starting high-dose steroids pending a temporal artery biopsy and rheumatology and ophthalmology opinions is the right thing to do.

4. A. Dapsone. The clinical appearance is pathognomonic of linear IgA disease and the first line drug of choice is dapsone. The rest of the choices are good therapeutic options that would be held in reserve if the patient failed to respond. Around 80% of patients will exhibit mucosal lesions, and whilst in many instances the aetiology is unknown, a number of medications have been identified as potential triggers, most notably vancomycin.

5. A. No further management. The histological appearances and HPV subtype along with the clinical picture is highly suggestive of focal epithelial hyperplasia (FEH) or Heck's disease. This is a self-limiting condition and as such requires no treatment beyond conservative excision of any troublesome lesions.

6. A. No further management. The histological features are diagnostic of a storiform collagenoma (or sclerotic fibroma) and excision is curative. It is a benign lesion and where isolated can be regarded as a single entity. Further lesions or other features (e.g. trichilemmomas) should prompt testing for mutation in the PTEN gene to screen for Cowden's disease.

7. D. *Bartonella henselae*. Cat scratch disease is exceedingly uncommon but an important differential for cervical lymphadenopathy, particularly in the face of non-specific histology. PCR testing for *Bartonella henselae* should be included in the series of tests for unexplained lymphadenopathy. *Borrelia burgdorferi* is the organism responsible for Lyme disease.

8. C. Verapamil. The history is entirely suggestive of cluster headaches, further supported by the increased incidence in males between the ages of 20 and 40. The frequency is less than would be expected from short-lasting unilateral neuralgiform headache with conjunctival injection and tearing (SUNCT), the lacrimation notwithstanding. Whilst triptans may be used as abortive treatment when an attack is underway, verapamil is recommended as a first line preventive agent.

9. B. It scavenges reactive oxygen species. A, C, D and E are all true but the comment about scavenging free radicals, (B) does not apply to pentoxyfylline, but rather applies to tocopherol (vitamin E). The work of Delanian and the PENTOCLO trial are useful points of reference for the potential impact of this combination on ORN.

10. C. Ruggiero. The Ruggiero system refers to medication-related osteonecrosis of the jaw (MRONJ), whilst the remaining options are all classification systems for osteoradionecrosis, the most recent being the staging system of Lyons et al. (2014).

11. A. No further management. Intravascular papillary endothelial hyperplasia (IPEH), also known as Masson's tumour or Masson's pseudoangiosarcoma, was first formally described in 1923. Initially presumed to be neoplastic in nature, IPEH is now recognized to be a benign, non-specific vascular lesion that arises as a reactive change resulting from the proliferation of endothelial cells in an organizing thrombus. Excision is curative.

12. A. Carbamazepine. International guidelines and Cochrane Reviews suggest that carbamazepine is the monotherapy of choice for trigeminal neuralgia, and indeed it is the only drug specifically licensed for its management in primary care. Oxcarbazepine is suggested where side-effects are poorly tolerated, with evidence existing for second line combination therapies including lamotrigine and baclofen, and gabapentin combined with ropivacaine.

13. B. Poorly differentiated SCC. Histology typically demonstrates intercellular bridging, frequent mitosis, and pleomorphism. Keratin pearls are seen on biopsy of differentiated SCC. Adenocarcinoma may resemble undifferentiated SCC, but intercellular bridging is not seen on biopsy. Adenoid cystic carcinoma is the most common malignant tumor of the minor salivary glands. Biopsy shows cylindrical epithelial masses that contain basophilic and pale-staining cells.

14. D. Hepatitis C virus infection increases the probability of it occurring. This area of biopsy-proven oral lichen planus (OLP) has undergone malignant transformation to oral squamous cell carcinoma (OSCC). A recent meta-analysis reported that 1.1% of OLP lesions progress into OSCC, with a higher incidence in smokers, alcohol users, and those infected with hepatitis C virus. Most commonly, malignant transformation occurs in erosive lesions and those localized on the tongue. Muñoz et al. identified that OSCC developed on pre-existing OLP lesions shows a higher rate of tumour recurrence compared to those with primary OSCC.

15. A. The patient should be reassured and reviewed in 6 months. The pigmentation likely represents smoker's melanosis and will resolve once the patient stops smoking. This may take a few years and relates to the amount of time they smoked for. The pigmentation is the result of increased melanin biosynthesis by the melanocytes. Biopsy is rarely required and only for isolated lesions where melanoma is a possibility. Although melanosis can occur with a large variety of drugs, changing the citalopram at this stage would not be warranted.

16. D. Corneal perforation. The clinical appearance and non-specific histology is suggestive of a drug-induced ulcer, most likely Nicorandil. This drug may cause painful ulceration anywhere in the gastrointestinal tract, eye, or the skin. Common additional side-effects of the drug include dizziness and headaches due to hypotension.

17. E. Nasal furuncle. Cavernous sinus thrombosis is a rare complication of common facial infections, most notably nasal furuncles (50%), sphenoidal or ethmoidal sinusitis (30%), and dental infections (10%). Patients with cavernous sinus thrombosis most commonly complain of fever, headache (50–90% of cases), peri-orbital swelling, or visual changes, such as photophobia, diplopia, or loss of vision.

18.   E. Fibrosis and granuloma formation.   This patient has erosive lichen planus. The central part of the lesion will likely demonstrate non-specific chronic inflammatory changes such lymphocytic infiltration replacing neutrophils. This will lead to fibrosis and granuloma formation. Only the periphery may show the classical histological features such as hydropic degeneration of the basal cells, scattered dyskeratotic keratinocytes (Civatte, colloid, hyaline, or cytoid bodies) along the epithelial interface, and a band-like, predominately T-lymphocyte infiltrate along the basement zone. Increased mitotic activity is a feature of SCC and not lichen planus.

19.   B. Treatment includes a carbonic anhydrase inhibitor.   This patient is likely to be suffering from migraines and not odontogenic pain. Topiramate is a commonly used drug to treat the effects. Sensitivity to light occurs in some cases of migraine but not all. Triptans or ergotamine may be used in those for whom simple pain medications are not effective. Caffeine may be added to the above.

20.   D. A treponemal test in conjunction with a non-treponemal test.   Both are required to make a presumptive diagnosis of tertiary syphilis, which occurs after 1 year of evolution in patients who have not received treatment in either primary or secondary stages. The characteristic destructive lesion of this phase, the gumma, may represent the chronic hypersensitivity reaction to the presence of spirochete. Dark-field microscopic examination is used to detect spirochetes in primary or secondary syphilis.

21.   C. Laser excision.   This is an inflammatory epulis and in a female patient pregnancy should be excluded as a causative factor. Otherwise either this is likely traumatic or there is an area of subgingival plaque. A necrotic tooth should be excluded with vitality testing. It is usually treated by scalpel excision and not by an ablative procedure such as a laser, because histology is required as occasional presentations of acute leukaemia have been described.

22.   D. The patient should be treated in a side room.   This patient has varicella zoster. Respiratory secretions are not usually a source of infection in shingles except in those with orofacial (trigeminal) disease and therefore a side room is indicated. This is a clinical diagnosis and routine PCR testing is not required. People with herpes zoster most commonly have a rash in one or two adjacent dermatomes. Acyclovir is given five times daily and so an oral dose would not be practicable. In addition, antiviral therapy is generally not given for patients presenting >72 hours after rash onset unless there is continued new vesicle formation or when there are cutaneous, motor, neurologic, or ocular complications.

23.   E. HIV.   Mucosal malignancy has been quoted as developing in the mucocutaneous variant of dyskeratosis congenita in 40% of cases, and in between 3 and 30% of cases of syphilis. Both Fanconi anaemia and HIV are pre-malignant conditions associated with human papilloma virus, but the latter only predisposes to SCC affecting the oropharynx and not the oral cavity.

24.   E. Severe dysplasia.   Cellular atypia and loss of normal maturation and stratification are signs of oral epithelial dysplasia. In the 3rd edition of the World Health Organization classification (El-Naggar et al, 2017) severe dysplasia is architectural disturbance present in more than two-thirds of the epithelium. In this classification, carcinoma in situ is now considered to be synonymous with severe dysplasia and the term carcinoma in situ is not used.

25. E. Cicatricial pemphigoid. This patient has desquamative gingivitis as part of cicatricial pemphigoid. Mucous membrane pemphigoid is a subtype of cicatricial pemphigoid when only the mucous membranes are affected. BP180 is a transmembrane collagen and a component of the hemidesmosomes of epithelial cells and may be detected on enzyme-linked immunosorbent assay (ELISA) testing.

26. D. Oral trazodone. The tongue appears grossly normal apart from some mild scalloping. This patient therefore likely has burning mouth syndrome, a term used to describe a group of symptoms for which no underlying cause can be found. Topical clonezapam has been shown in studies to have similar efficacy to oral clonezapam. A placebo-controlled, double-blind study by Tammiala-Salonen and Forssell (1999) did not show any benefit from treatment with the serotoninergic antidepressant trazodone.

27. B. Skin pigmentation is likely. This patient has dyskeratosis congenita, an inherited disease due to severe shortening of telomeres. It is characterized by the triad of skin pigmentation, nail dystrophy, and oral leukoplakia. It results in bone marrow failure and a predisposition to a multitude of malignancies. Thirty percent of leukoplakia lesions in such patients undergo malignant transformation.

28. C. Haemoglobin. This patient likely has necrotizing fasciitis. This is a clinical diagnosis, although a score of score >6 has PPV of 92% of having necrotizing fasciitis according to the Laboratory Risk Indicator for Necrotizing Fasciitis (LRINEC) scoring system. This comprises a CRP ≥150 (4 points), white blood cells (WBCs) >25 (2 points), haemoglobin <11 (2 points), sodium <135 (2 points), creatinine >141 (2 points), and glucose >10 (1 point). In a diabetic patient with renal failure, the latter two parameters would be of limited use with this system. Chronic renal failure also causes a drop in haemoglobin.

29. D. Surgical vermilionectomy. Patients with diffuse actinic cheilitis may benefit from topical fluorouracil or imiquimod. Photodynamic therapy has also been described. Patients with severe diffuse actinic cheilitis without evidence of high-grade dysplasia or cancer on biopsy should be treated with ablation with carbon dioxide (CO_2) or Er:YAG laser. Vermilionectomy ensures the histopathologic examination of the entire vermilion and is the treatment of choice for actinic cheilitis with severe dysplasia on biopsy.

30. E. Post-operative hypophosphataemia or hypomagnesaemia should instigate slowing of NG feeding. This patient is at risk of refeeding syndrome and requires regular monitoring for potassium, magnesium, calcium, and phosphate levels. Deficiencies should be treated with intravenous supplementation and NG feeding slowed (but not stopped). According to the British Society of Gastroenterology 'Guidelines for enteral feeding in adult hospital patients', a PEG is only required if enteral feeding is predicted to last longer than 4 weeks, which in this scenario is unlikely. Post-operative NG feeding in head and neck cancer patients should be instigated within 24 hours. The Duke University Pre-Operative Nutrition Score assessment as highlighted by Gillis and Wischmeyer (2019) requires measurement of body mass index, albumin, and vitamin D.

References

Delanian S, Depondt J, Lafaix JL (2005). Major healing of refractory osteoradionecrosis after treatment combining pentoxifylline and tocopherol: a phase II trial. *Head Neck* **27**(2):114–123.

Delanian S, Chatel C, Porcher R, et al (2011). Complete restoration of refractory mandibular osteoradionecrosis by prolonged treatment with a pentoxyfylline-tocopherol-clodronate combination (PENTOCLO): a phase II trial. *International Journal of Radiation Oncology, Biology, Physics* **80**(3):832–839.

El-Naggar AK, Chan JK, Grandis JR, et al (2017). *WHO Classification of Head and Neck Tumours 4th Edition*. International Agency for Research on Cancer (IARC) Press.

Gillis C, Wischmeyer PE (2019). Pre-operative nutrition and the elective surgical patient: why, how and what? *Anaesthesia* **74**(S1):27–35.

Lyons A, Osher J, Warner E, et al (2014). Osteoradionecrosis: a review of current concepts in defining extent of the disease and a new classification proposal. *British Journal of Oral and Maxillofacial Surgery* **52**(3):392–395.

Muñoz AA, Haddad RI, Woo SB, Bhattacharyya N (2016). Behaviour of oral squamous cell carcinoma in subjects with prior lichen planus. *Otolaryngology–Head and Neck Surgery* **136**(3):401–404.

Stroud M, Duncan H, Nightingale J, British Society of Gastroenterology (2003). Guidelines for enteral feeding in adult hospital patients. *Gut* **52** (Suppl 7):vii1–vii12.

Tammiala-Salonen T, Forssell H (1999). Trazodone in burning mouth pain: a placebo-controlled, double-blind study. *Journal of Orofacial Pain* **13**(2):83–88.

1. **You are asked to see a child in the craniofacial clinic who has recently been adopted from overseas. They have micrognathia but are otherwise phenotypically normal. Genetic testing has detected an abnormality of the TCOF1 gene. Which one of the following is the *least* common presentation of this syndrome?**
   A. Symmetrical
   B. Parotid hyperplasia
   C. Hypertelorism
   D. Sensorineural hearing loss
   E. Cleft palate

2. **Which of the following regarding vascular anomalies is false?**
   A. A pyogenic granuloma is a benign vascular tumour
   B. An arteriovenous fistula is a high-flow vascular malformation
   C. A congenital haemangioma may not involute
   D. A Kaposi sarcoma is a malignant vascular tumour
   E. Angiosarcoma may occur after radiation exposure

3. **A dentist has referred an 8-year-old boy with generalized advanced caries. A panoramic radiograph demonstrates a small condyle and ramus but the sigmoid notch is visible. They have a partially formed ear, for which they are awaiting assessment. Which of the following is true?**
   A. Treatment of the mandible should be with a costochondral graft if normal mouth opening is present
   B. Autologous ear reconstruction is performed when the patient has stopped growing
   C. Treatment timing is guided by the presence of a maxillary cant
   D. Facial reanimation should be accomplished using a one-stage cross-face nerve graft
   E. Structural fat grafts will demonstrate less resorption than dermal fat grafts

4. **You are asked to review the computed tomography (CT) scan of a 14-year-old girl who was hit in the head accidently by a tennis racket. She has been experiencing headaches ever since. The scan demonstrates displacement of the cerebellar tonsils through the foramen magnum. Which of the following is true?**
    A. The headaches are due to an underlying craniofacial condition
    B. The patient requires surgery to relieve raised intracranial pressure
    C. The patient is at risk of developing symptoms later in life
    D. Developmental delay is a common presentation of this condition
    E. The patient requires further imaging with magnetic resonance (MR)

5. **You are reviewing the imaging of a lump on the tongue of a 10-year-old in clinic. The lesion demonstrates phleboliths, flow voids, and cysts of approximately 2 cm. Which of the following is true?**
    A. Excision is the preferred treatment modality
    B. Ultrasound (US) alone is sufficient imaging to proceed for excision
    C. The size of the lump on examination determines the need for tracheostomy
    D. These lesions often have a red speckled appearance
    E. Doxycycline is an effective treatment of this condition

6. **You are reviewing the results of a CT scan in the craniofacial clinic. Which condition is related to only a single suture?**
    A. Scaphocephaly
    B. Oxycephaly
    C. Cloverleaf skull
    D. Positional plagiocephaly
    E. Brachycephaly

7. **Which of the following statements regarding midface distraction osteogenesis in a syndromic patient is true?**
    A. Midface advancement without mandibular surgery may allow for tracheostomy decannulation
    B. Subcranial Le Fort III osteotomy is one that includes a monobloc
    C. Le Fort I and III procedures may use distraction but a Le Fort II does not
    D. A Le Fort III is used in midface hypoplasia with an acceptable position of the zygomatic complex and orbits
    E. It is usually performed at approximately 3 years old

8. **You are removing a 12-mm cancerous skin lesion of a 40-year-old patient. He has a prominent forehead and has been a long-term patient of yours for similar lesions and attends with his 10-year-old daughter. Which of the following is true?**

A. His daughter has a 25% chance of inheriting this condition
B. The patient will have bifid ribs
C. He requires serial panoramic radiographic monitoring
D. The lesion should be excised with a 3-mm margin
E. This condition will not affect his daughter's fertility

9. **You receive an urgent referral for assessment of a pulsatile mass on the lateral tongue of a 25-year-old woman, that has grown over the last few months, as shown in Figure 10.1. The lesion bleeds spontaneously and is painful. Which of the following is true?**

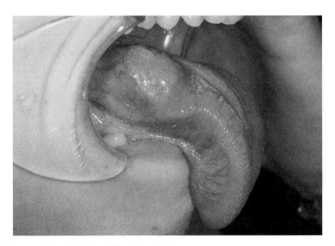

Figure 10.1 Mass on the right lateral border of the tongue.

A. The lesion will appear white on a T2-weighted MR image
B. Treatment should include excision of both inflow and outflow vessels
C. The lesion is treated through endovascular techniques at the time of surgery
D. The lesion is classified as grade two according to Schobinger
E. Ulceration is unlikely

10. **A patient with a longstanding enlargement of their lip underwent an injection into the lip 5 days ago. Initially no additional swelling was seen, but today the patient presents to the emergency department with appearance shown in Figure 10.2. Which of the following is the most appropriate management?**

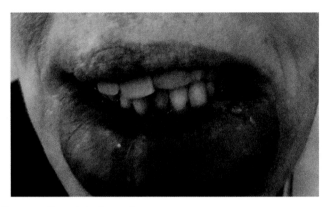

Figure 10.2 Gross swelling of the lower lip.

   A. Admission for intravenous antibiotics
   B. Admission for surgical drainage
   C. Discharge with oral antibiotics
   D. Assessment with US
   E. Reassurance

11. **This patient shown in Figure 10.3 is awaiting surgery. Their mouth opening is one finger width with a prominent maxillary cant. Which of the following is true?**
   A. They have a class III classification according to Pruzansky
   B. Sagittal split osteotomy on the right side is indicated
   C. Distraction osteogenesis is indicated
   D. Contemporaneous joint replacement is not indicated
   E. The patient has a number eight facial cleft

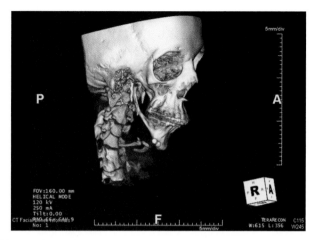

Figure 10.3 CT scan of a patient preoperatively awaiting corrective surgery.

12. A 9-month-old baby is brought into clinic by her foster parents with a hand shown in Figure 10.4. No information is known about her birth parents, but genetic testing has demonstrated a mutation of the FGFr2 gene. Which of the following is true?

A. Cognitive function is normally impaired

B. The baby's father was most likely a carrier for the genetic mutation

C. Bone abnormalities are restricted to the hands and feet

D. Two fused digits are most common

E. Digit reconstruction is undertaken at approximately 1 year of age

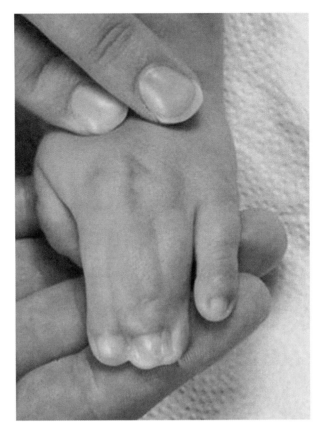

Figure 10.4 Appearance of the hand of a 9-month-old baby awaiting surgery.

13. **This child with the radiograph shown in Figure 10.5 presents with a 6-month history of facial swelling, unresponsive to antibiotics. Biopsy demonstrates the presence of copious amounts of osteoid. Which of the following is true?**

    A. This child is at least 7 years old
    B. Tooth mobility is a rare presentation
    C. Ewing's sarcoma is the most likely cause
    D. This pathology is more common in the facial bones than the long bones
    E. The primary treatment modality is chemotherapy

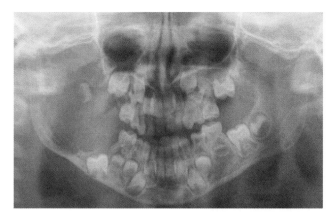

Figure 10.5 OPG radiograph taken in a child with unilateral facial swelling.

14. **You review this baby's head shape, as shown in Figure 10.6, in clinic due to concerns from the parents. The baby's ear is pushed further forwards on the right side compared to the left. Which of the following is true?**

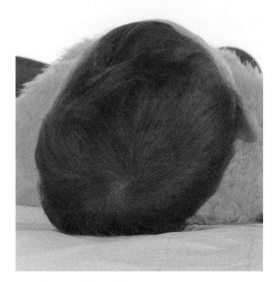

Figure 10.6 Appearance of the skull in a child on presentation.

A. Compensatory contralateral anterior displacement of the cheek may occur
B. The cranial base will be tilted
C. Lambdoid synostosis is the most likely diagnosis
D. The condition should be treated first by helmet therapy
E. The parents should continue to lie the baby on his or her back at night

15. **A patient with the radiograph shown in Figure 10.7 has a mutation of the RUNX2 gene. Which of the following are true?**

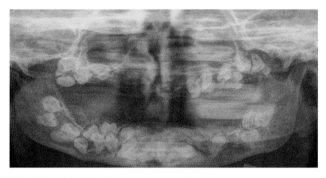

Figure 10.7 OPG radiograph of patient on presentation.

    A. Multiple supernumerary teeth are most commonly non-syndromic
    B. Complete absence of the clavicles can occur
    C. Crowding is exacerbated by mandibular hypoplasia
    D. Delayed or failed closure of the anterior fontanelle may occur
    E. A prominent metopic suture is likely present

16. **A 5-year-old child presents with a midline neck swelling that moves on swallowing. Which of the following is true of a patient of this age?**
    A. This age is an unusual presentation for this type of pathology
    B. This most likely represents a branchial cleft anomaly
    C. This most likely represents ectopic thyroid tissue
    D. It most commonly presents with pain
    E. The epithelial lining of the swelling will resemble acinar cells

17. **A baby with Treacher Collins syndrome and a facial cleft presents to the craniofacial clinic. Which of the following is false?**
    A. The ipsilateral ear will commonly be affected
    B. This cleft is also associated with craniofacial microsomia (CFM)
    C. This is most likely a Tessier number 7 facial cleft
    D. The masseter muscle is rarely affected
    E. The cleft is due to failed fusion of the maxillary and zygomatic prominences in utero

18. **A 2-year-old girl returns to the joint craniofacial clinic following failed extubation of her tracheostomy. Her phenotype includes maxillary hypoplasia and a cleft palate. You notice a bone-anchored hearing aid. Which of the following is true of her syndrome?**

A. It can be due to a defect in the treacle gene

B. It most commonly occurs due to spontaneous mutations

C. It displays autosomal recessive inheritance when the TCOF1 gene is mutated

D. It is due to a mutation in the treacle gene

E. It displays autosomal dominant inheritance when the POLR1D gene is mutated

19. **A review of a CT scan in a 30-year-old man demonstrates three bone radiodense masses in the mandible and skull. He recently underwent prophylactic proctocolectomy. Which of the following is true?**

A. The patient will have deletion of the APC gene

B. Genetic testing should be undertaken at birth

C. Cancer surveillance must begin at skeletal maturity

D. These lesions likely represent osteoblastomas

E. Dermoid cysts will be present affecting the face

20. **Which of the following are true of raised intracranial pressure associated with non- syndromic craniosynostosis?**

A. Brain volume expansion in the normally developing child doubles in the first 2 years of life

B. It commonly occurs following sagittal and lambdoid suture synostosis

C. Surgery is indicated due to raised intracranial pressure when it exceeds 10 mmHg

D. Symptoms include headaches, visual disturbances, and deafness

E. It commonly occurs with a Chiari type 1 malformation leading to papilloedema

1. D. Sensorineural hearing loss. TCOF 1, POLR1C, and POLR1D are the genes most commonly responsible for Treacher Collins syndrome. The phenotype of Treacher Collins is a bilateral symmetrical one in which the parotid glands demonstrate aplasia or hypoplasia. Hearing loss is conductive.

2. D. Kaposi sarcoma is a malignant vascular tumour. According to the 2018 International Society for the Study of Vascular Anomalies (ISSVA) classification for vascular anomalies, a Kaposi sarcoma is a locally aggressive or borderline vascular tumour. Angiosarcoma is a rare but aggressive malignant vascular tumour often associated with prior radiotherapy.

3. C. Treatment timing is guided by the presence of a maxillary cant. CFM involves an absence or underdevelopment of structures that arise from the first and second pharyngeal arches, such as the mandible, maxilla, ear, facial soft tissue and muscles, and the facial nerve. Facial reanimation can also be accomplished using a two-stage approach with a cross-face nerve graft and muscle-free flap. Soft tissue augmentation with dermal fat grafts is often more advantageous than structural fat grafts, as the latter can demonstrate resorption of 30–80% of the injected fat, depending on location.

4. C. The patient is at risk of developing symptoms later in life. CT scan appearance is in keeping with a type 1 Chiari malformation. It is usually first noticed in adolescence or adulthood, often by accident during an examination for another condition. Adolescents and adults who have Chiari type 1 malformation but no symptoms initially may develop signs of the disorder later in life.

5. E. Doxycycline is effective treatment of this condition. This lesion likely represents a low flow venous or mixed lymph–venous malformation. Low flow lesions are treated by sclerotherapy but require both US and MR to determine their full extent and examination is often misleading. Doxycycline is as effective as Sodium Tetradecyl Sulphate for macro cystic lesions, which are 2 cm or greater. A red speckled appearance generally represents a micro cystic lesion.

6. A. Scaphocephaly. This is due to isolated sagittal synostosis. Oxycephaly is premature closure of all sutures. Cloverleaf skull is synostosis involving the coronal, sagittal, and lambdoid sutures. Brachycephaly is bicoronal synostosis.

7. A. Midface advancement without mandibular surgery may allow for tracheostomy decannulation. A Le Fort II is used in midface hypoplasia with an acceptable position of the zygomatic complex and orbits. A subcranial Le Fort III osteotomy can be converted to a monobloc procedure if a retrusive midface is present. Midface distraction is often done when children are 8–10 years old; however, if breathing is a problem it may be performed as young as 3 years old.

8. E. This condition will not affect his daughter's fertility. The patient has Gorlin's syndrome, which has autosomal dominant inheritance. Odontogenic keratocysts (OKC), previously known as keratocystic odontogenic tumours, do not develop in humans over 30 years old. Only 60% have bifid ribs. Females can develop fibromas, but these do not affect fertility.

9. A. The lesion will appear white on a T2-weighted MR image. In the Schobinger classification of arteriovenous malformations (AVMs), pulsatility and expansion indicate grade 2. Spontaneous bleeding indicates grade 3 and is often accompanied by ulceration. Lesions at this stage generally require treatment, which usually involves embolization followed by surgery within a few days. To prevent recurrence, surgery must excise the lesion 'nidus' which acts as an angiogenic centre.

10. E. Reassurance. This is an expected complication and reassurance is required. This patient has likely been treated with bleomycin, which induces swelling that may start 5 days later.

11. A. They have a class III classification according to Pruzansky. This is because the glenoid fossa is totally absent, the ramus is grossly distorted, and there is absence of joint function. This patient has hemifacial (craniofacial) microsomia and a number 7 facial cleft according to the Tessier classification. This patient is in fixed orthodontics, likely awaiting bimaxillary orthognathic surgery. Distraction osteogenesis is not indicated.

12. E. Digit reconstruction is undertaken at approximately 1 year of age. This patient has Apert syndrome, in which there is a spectrum of normal to moderately disabled cognitive function. Some people with Apert syndrome have abnormalities in the bones of the elbows or shoulders. Inheritance may be autosomal dominant, but most new cases are sporadic mutations of the FGFr2 gene. Most commonly, three digits on each hand and foot are fused together. Operative surgical release of digits is performed at approximately 1 year of age and digit reconstruction performed 6 months later to convert the central three digits into two digits.

13. A. This child is at least 7 years old. This is most likely an osteosarcoma. The observation of osteoid is key for the diagnosis of osteosarcoma, the most common primary bony malignancy in the mandible. These cases are rare and most commonly are mistaken as dental infections. The most common presenting symptoms are swelling and pain. Osteosarcoma occurs most frequently in the lower long bones, with the maxilla and mandible representing only about 7% of cases. Treatment is by surgery with contemporaneous reconstruction, but adjuvant chemotherapy has been shown to improve survival. The adult lateral incisors are fully erupted, indicating that the patient is at least 7 years old.

14. E. The parents should continue to lie the baby on his or her back at night. This patient has positional plagiocephaly because there is both frontal and occipitoparietal flattening. Ipsilateral anterior displacement of the forehead and cheek may occur. The differential diagnoses include unicoronal or lambdoid synostosis, but the ear would be set back relatively on the affected side. Frequent rotation of the child's head would be the first recommendation. Parents should be advised to continue placing their baby on his or her back to sleep, even if the child has positional plagiocephaly.

15. D. Delayed or failed closure of the anterior fontanel. This patient has cleidocranial dysplasia. Non-syndromic multiple supernumerary teeth are very rare, with the incidence of <1%. One or both clavicles can be partly missing, leaving only the medial part of the bone. Relative pseudoprognathism of the mandible occurs due to hypoplasia of the maxilla. The skull usually demonstrates calvarial thickening in the supraorbital ridge, and a persistent metopic suture.

16. E. The epithelial lining of the swelling will resemble acinar cells . This child likely has a thyroglossal duct cyst, of which 90% present before 10 years old. Most are in the midline, or just to one side of it. They are usually slow-growing painless fluctuant swellings unless they become infected. The cysts can occur anywhere along the course of the thyroglossal duct from the foramen caecum to the thyroid gland: suprahyoid (20–25%), level of hyoid bone (15–50%), and infrahyoid (25–65%). The cystic epithelial lining if found near the tongue will be stratified squamous epithelium, but those found in the neck are lined with cells similar to thyroidal acinar epithelium.

17. E. The cleft is due to failed fusion of the maxillary and zygomatic prominences in utero. This is false. It is due to failed fusion of the maxillary and mandibular prominences in utero and is termed a number 7 cleft by the Tessier system. Tessier believed that the cleft is centred in the region of the zygomaticotemporal suture and it is sometimes termed a zygomaticotemporal cleft. This cleft is seen in CFM, and in Treacher Collins syndrome clefts of number 6 and number 8 can also occur. The cleft begins at the oral commissure and varies from a mild broadening of the oral commissure with a pre-auricular skin tag to a complete fissure extending towards a microtic ear. Typically, the cleft does not extend beyond the anterior border of the masseter.

18. B. It most commonly occurs due to spontaneous mutations. Genetics and inheritance of craniofacial conditions have been a recurring theme in the FRCS examination. This patient likely has Treacher Collins syndrome, of which about 60% of cases occur from new mutations. The midface hypoplasia differentiates the presentation from Pierre Robin sequence. When Treacher Collins results from mutations in the TCOF1 gene it is considered an autosomal dominant condition and when it results from mutations in the POLR1D gene it is considered autosomal recessive inheritance. The TCOF1 gene carries instructions that encode a protein known as treacle.

19. A. The patient will have deletion of the APC gene. This patient has Gardner syndrome. Associations include increased risk of recurrent osteomas and epidermoid cysts. Some patients who have familial adenomatous polyposis undergo proctocolectomy due to the increased risk of colorectal cancer. Colon screening for those at risk for Gardner syndrome begins as early as age 10 years old. Carrier testing for at-risk relatives and pre-natal testing are possible if the disease-causing mutation in the family is known.

20. B. It commonly occurs following sagittal and lambdoid suture synostosis. Brain volume expansion in the normally developing child almost triples during the first year of life. Surgery is indicated due to raised intracranial pressure (when it exceeds 15 mmHg). Symptoms of raised intracranial pressure include headaches, visual disturbances, and ringing in the ears. Raised intracranial pressure if untreated may lead to papilloedema, but it is rarely due to a Chiari type 1 malformation.

Reference

International Society for the Study of Vascular Anomalies (ISSVA) classification for vascular anomalies. Approved at the 20th ISSVA Workshop, Melbourne, April 2014, last revision May 2018. Accessible at: https://www.issva.org/UserFiles/file/ISSVA-Classification-2018.pdf

1. **You are planning to treat a 12-month-old patient with a cleft palate. Which of the following is *not* a goal of this procedure?**

   A. Separation of the oral and nasal cavities

   B. Creation of a competent velopharyngeal (VP) valve for swallowing and speech

   C. Preservation of midface growth

   D. Reduction in intraoral breath pressure

   E. Promotion of development of a functional occlusion

2. **Which of the following is true of cleft lip and palate?**

   A. An incomplete cleft lip will rarely affect the nasal sill

   B. This condition is present in 1:500 live births in the UK

   C. It requires an immediate referral at birth to the cleft team to enable feeding

   D. Hearing loss is treated with a bone-anchored hearing aid

   E. A bone graft provides support for the teeth either side of the cleft

3. **A patient presents with an underdeveloped orbit, external ear, and facial cleft. This cleft results from failure in fusion of which structures?**

   A. Failure of fusion of the maxillary prominence with the medial nasal prominence

   B. Maxillary and mandibular processes

   C. Left and right mandibular processes

   D. Maxillary and frontonasal processes

   E. Mandibular and hyoid arches

4. **You review a cleft palate patient undergoing surgical treatment as shown in the radiograph (Figure 11.1) and notice a 3-mm midline shift. Which of the following interventions is recommended?**

   A. Continue as planned

   B. Reposition fixators

   C. Provide patient education

   D. Reosteotomize the maxilla

   E. Provide post-surgical orthodontics

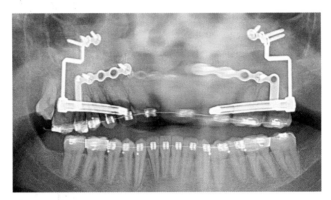

Figure 11.1 OPG radiograph of a cleft patient in orthodontic appliances.

5. **The previously treated cleft palate patient shown in Figure 11.2 complains of occasional nasal regurgitation of fluids but is otherwise asymptomatic. Which is most correct about this defect?**

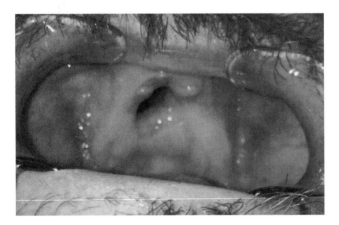

Figure 11.2 Palatal fistula in an adult cleft patient.

    A. The Pittsburg system is commonly used to grade severity
    B. It is most commonly repaired using a tongue flap
    C. A fistulogram may guide the need for treatment
    D. A posterior pharyngeal flap can be used for repair
    E. It is more likely to have been due to a Veau IV cleft than a Veau I

6. **Which of the following may alter your technique in performing a Le Fort I osteotomy in cleft patients?**

A. Nasomaxillary hypoplasia
B. Large anteroposterior movement
C. Previous pharyngeal flap
D. United lesser segment
E. Absent velopharyngeal (VP) insufficiency

7. **Which of the following is correct regarding the muscles in achieving VP closure?**

A. The superior pharyngeal constrictor muscles move the posterior pharyngeal wall inferiorly
B. The levator palatini pulls the soft palate posteriorly
C. The palatopharyngeus muscles pull the soft palate superiorly
D. The musculus uvulae pulls the uvula apart
E. The superior pharyngeal constrictor muscles pull the lateral pharyngeal walls superiorly

8. **Which of the following is not true of the Tennison–Randall cleft lip reconstruction technique?**

A. It relies upon rigid geometric design rather than surgeon experience
B. It is particularly useful for wide clefts with severe vertical deficiency
C. It may produce a lip that is too long
D. Closure does not follow the borders of anatomic subunits
E. It uses a back-cut filled by a medially based triangular flap

9. **The rationale for alveolar bone grafting in a 9-year-old patient includes all of the below except:**

A. Enabling the maxillary canines to erupt
B. Closure of an oro-antral fistula
C. Facilitating orthodontic alignment of the teeth
D. Fusing the maxilla into a single segment for a future osteotomy
E. Creating support for the nose (alar base) and lip

10. **The patient shown in Figure 11.3 is awaiting surgery on her nose. Which of the following is true?**

A. This is best carried out as a closed procedure to preserve vascularity
B. It is generally carried out at the same time as orthognathic surgery
C. It is rarely required
D. Septorhinoplasty is usually performed
E. A supplementary bone strut is rarely required

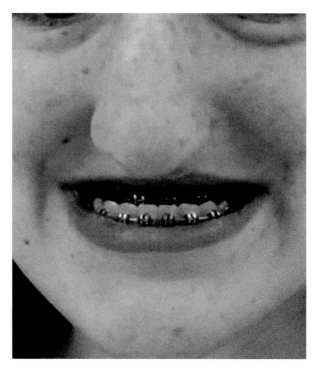

Figure 11.3 A patient in orthodontic appliances awaiting surgery on her nose.

11. **Which of the following is false about primary rhinoplasty at the time of cleft lip surgery?**
    A. It closes the nasal floor and sill
    B. It restricts nasal growth
    C. It repositions the alar bases anteriorly, superiorly, and medially
    D. It creates an asymmetrical contour of the lower lateral cartilages
    E. It reduces tip projection

12. **Regarding resonance disorders in cleft patients, which of the following is true?**
    A. Nearly all patients get normal speech resonance and nasal emission following surgery
    B. Resonance disorders are usually due to mislearning
    C. Most vowels and consonants in the English language are nasal
    D. Resonance is a function of airflow
    E. The VP valve is the main determinant of speech resonance

13. You review an 8-year-old in combined cleft clinic that has been lost to follow-up for a number of years. Examination demonstrates a symptomatic oronasal fistula (ONF) in the posterior palate. Which of the following is false?

A. The patient may have hypernasality and nasal emission
B. They will likely have difficulty in articulating the consonants d and t
C. The ONF was most likely due to an original repair that was placed under too much tension
D. Infection is a rare cause of failure in primary palatal repair in children
E. The ONF is likely to be larger than 5 mm

14. Which of the following features of a cleft lip is not correct?

A. Cupid's bow is rotated towards the cleft side
B. The philtral column is shorter on the cleft side
C. The nasal tip is flat and deflected to the cleft side
D. The columella on the cleft side is shortened
E. A wide alveolar cleft may be present

15. Which of the following is false about velopharyngeal dysfunction (VPD)?

A. VPD occurs when the valve does not close consistently
B. VPD occurs when the valve does not close completely
C. The valve comprises the velum, lateral pharyngeal walls, and posterior pharyngeal wall
D. Velopharyngeal valve insufficiency is the most common cause of VPD
E. Cleft palate is a cause of velopharyngeal valve incompetence

1. D. Reduction in intraoral breath pressure. In the UK cleft palate repair is generally performed when children are approximately 12 months old. The main goal of surgery is to improve the long-term quality of speech, with secondary goals including promoting development of the occlusion and eustachian tube function. The inability to generate intraoral breath pressure due to nasal air emission manifests as articulation difficulties, particularly consonant weakness.

2. E. A bone graft provides support for the teeth either side of the cleft. In addition to its primary role in facilitating eruption of the canine tooth, the graft supports in particular the lateral incisor tooth. An incomplete cleft lip will not affect the nasal sill as it does not involve the full height of the lip. Feeding advice is provided on the ward after birth and formal referral by the paediatric team is generally made after a few weeks. Hearing loss is conductive due to abnormal eustachian tube anatomy causing recurrent otitis media.

3. B. Maxillary and mandibular processes. Lateral facial clefts, producing macrostomia, result from failure of the maxillary and mandibular prominences to fuse at the lateral commissure. This is classified by the Tessier system as a number 7 facial cleft.

4. D. Reosteotomize the maxilla. This patient with a bilateral cleft is at the start of treatment with only 3–5 mm of movement. Fixation appears sound and correctly positioned. Symmetrical movement would be expected at this stage and most likely represents incomplete separation of the left-sided fragment, which should be re-osteotomized.

5. E. It is more likely to have been due to a Veau IV cleft than a Veau I. The Pittsburg system is used to describe fistula position, in which this is a class IV. No consensus exists as to the best type of repair. Techniques include elevation of mucoperiosteal flaps with pushback, labial mucosal flap, buccal myomucosal flap, facial artery musculomucosal (FAMM) flap, tongue flap, and free tissue transfer. A posterior pharyngeal flap is used for type III defects and only if VPD is present. Patients with a Veau IV cleft (complete bilateral soft, hard, and/or lip and alveolar ridge cleft) are the most prone to develop an oronasal fistula.

6. C. Previous pharyngeal flap. Although a pharyngeal flap is not a limiting factor when performing a maxillary advancement, the pedicle may produce caudal tension and should be reinserted in a higher position at the time of osteotomy. Patients with established VP insufficiency may worsen post advancement, and simultaneous or secondary pharyngoplasty should be considered. Modifications of the Le Fort I technique were developed to enable differential movement of the maxillary segments and closure of dental gaps in both unilateral and bilateral clefts and simultaneous grafting of the alveolar clefts. When nasomaxillary hypoplasia is present, proposed a Le Fort II osteotomy is performed, as first recommended by Henderson and Jackson.

7. B. The levator palatini pulls the soft palate posteriorly. The levator palatini muscles are the most important for achieving VP closure and pull the middle third of the soft palate superiorly and posteriorly. The paired palatopharyngeus muscles pull the soft palate posteriorly. The musculus uvulae causes the uvula to thicken centrally with contraction. The superior pharyngeal constrictor muscles move the lateral pharyngeal walls medially or the posterior pharyngeal wall anteriorly with contraction.

8. E. It uses a back-cut filled by a medially based triangular flap. This is false. The Tennison–Randall technique involves a back-cut that extends from the cleft cupid's bow peak towards the centre of the philtrum that is filled by a laterally based triangular flap whose width is the measured deficiency in lip height.

9. B. Closure of an oro-antral fistula. This is false. In the UK a secondary alveolar bone graft is performed at approximately 9 years old. Other indications include improving periodontal health and providing increased bony support to teeth adjacent to the cleft. This will enable the canine to erupt, and by this point maxillary growth is almost complete so it should not interfere with it.

10. D. Septorhinoplasty is usually performed. Unlike primary rhinoplasty, secondary cleft rhinoplasty is best carried out as an open procedure and should be carried out after orthognathic surgery. Secondary rhinoplasty is commonly required as clefts often involve the nose and is best carried out after growth is complete. A septorhinoplasty is commonly performed and often requires a cartilaginous nasal strut.

11. B. It restricts nasal growth. This is false. The majority of cleft surgeons have now incorporated primary rhinoplasty into their practice with excellent results. The latest evidence suggests that primary rhinoplasty at the time of cleft lip surgery does not impair nasal growth.

12. E. The VP valve is the main determinant of speech resonance. A systematic review by de Blacam et al. (2018) demonstrated that 71% of patients attained normal speech resonance and 65% attained normal nasal emission. Resonance disorders can result from structural or functional causes and occasionally are due to mislearning. Most vowels and vocalic consonants in the English language are predominantly oral. Resonance is a function of sound and not airflow.

13. B. They will likely have difficulty in articulating the consonants d and t. This is false as the defect is posterior. Only those oronasal fistulas that are anterior will result in misarticulation of tongue-tip sounds. Tongue-tip elevation is an oral motor skill necessary to say certain speech sounds (t, d, n, l, s, and z). Larger ONFs (>5 mm) are more likely to be symptomatic. Symptoms include patient will likely have hypernasality, nasal emission, and compensatory articulation. ONF develops most commonly because of repair under tension and in some cases, especially in adults, as a result of post-operative infection.

14. C. The nasal tip is flat and deflected to the cleft side. This is false. In fact, the nasal tip is flat and deflected to the non-cleft side. Cupid's bow is upwardly rotated towards the cleft side. Depending on the involvement of the alveolus, it may range from intact to a wide alveolar cleft.

15. E. Cleft palate is a cause of VP incompetence. This is false. Cleft palate is a cause of VP insufficiency and not incompetence. The VP valve comprises the velum, lateral pharyngeal walls, and posterior pharyngeal wall. VPD occurs when the VP valve does not close consistently or completely during the production of oral sounds. It is used as a general term that encompasses disorders of any of the three basic components of VP function, namely structure (insufficiency), function (incompetence), and learning.

References

de Blacam C, Smith S, Orr D (2018). Surgery for Velopharyngeal Dysfunction: A Systematic Review of Interventions and Outcomes. *The Cleft Palate-Craniofacial Journal* **55**(3):405–422.

Henderson D, Jackson IT (1973). Nasomaxillary Hypoplasis—the Lefort II osteotomy. *British Journal of Oral Surgery* **11**(2):77–93.

1. **A 24-year-old woman with Crohn's disease has had multiple episodes of recurrent pericoronitis related to her horizontally impacted lower right third molar. Her inflammatory bowel disease is well controlled with azathioprine. On an orthopantomogram (OPG), the 'white line' of the inferior alveolar nerve canal appears interrupted by the third molar roots. Her contralateral third molar shows similar appearances but has been asymptomatic. What is the next most appropriate management?**
   A. Removal of the right third molar
   B. Removal of the bilateral lower third molars
   C. Coronectomy of the lower right third molars
   D. No treatment (watchful waiting)
   E. Cone beam computed tomography (CBCT) scan

2. **An apicectomy of an upper central incisor is performed and at the time of placing the root-end filling, moisture control proves difficult. Which would be the filling material of choice?**
   A. Reinforced zinc oxide eugenol cement
   B. Ethoxybenzoic acid
   C. Amalgam
   D. Mineral trioxide aggregate (MTA)
   E. Glass ionomer cement (GIC)

3. **A patient with Ludwig's angina secondary to a carious lower right second molar is brought in to the resuscitation bay of the emergency department. His oxygen saturations quickly plummet and a senior registrar in anaesthetics makes two attempts to intubate the patient but is unable to achieve an airway. What is the next step in management?**
   A. Laryngeal mask airway (LMA™)
   B. Needle cricothyroidotomy
   C. Surgical cricothyroidotomy
   D. Percutaneous tracheostomy
   E. Surgical tracheostomy

4. **Q7. A 24-year-old man undergoes surgical removal of a disto-angular impacted lower left third molar. Which technique is likely to yield the lowest rates of permanent lingual nerve injury?**

    A. No lingual retraction
    B. Lingual split technique
    C. Lingual retraction with a repurposed retractor
    D. Lingual retraction with a purpose-built retractor
    E. Benex® extraction system

5. **A 25-year-old woman has removal of a disto-angular lower left third molar carried out. Subsequent to this she notices a 75% reduction in sensation and loss of taste on the ipsilateral side of her tongue. How soon after the initial surgery should exploratory surgery be undertaken to optimize chances of recovery (if this is felt to be warranted and mutually agreed upon with the patient)?**

    A. Within 1 week
    B. Within 1 month
    C. Within 3 months
    D. Within 6 months
    E. Within 1 year

6. **Two years after surgery to remove an impacted lower third molar, a 35-year-old woman is still experiencing profound numbness of the right side of her lower lip and chin, although she denies any neuropathic pain or allodynia. She finds that she actively avoids social engagements that involve eating with friends. What treatment modality could be offered to her?**

    A. Cognitive behavioural therapy (CBT)
    B. Amitriptyline
    C. Pregabalin
    D. External neurolysis +/− repair of the right inferior alveolar nerve
    E. Topical capsaicin

7. **Which of the following nerves are *not* at risk of injury during autogenous bone graft harvest from the anterior iliac crest?**

    A. Lateral cutaneous branch of the subcostal nerve
    B. Lateral cutaneous branch of the iliohypogastric nerve
    C. Lateral femoral cutaneous nerve
    D. Femoral nerve
    E. Superior cluneal nerve

8. **A 16-year-old boy suffers an avulsion injury of his central incisor, which is kept dry in a tissue for 90 minutes prior to his arrival in the emergency department. Which of the following is the ideal course of management?**
    A. Avoid replanting the tooth
    B. Replant the tooth and splint with a rigid splint for up to 14 days
    C. Replant the tooth and splint with a flexible splint for up to 14 days
    D. Replant the tooth and advise that the dentist should monitor the tooth clinically and radiographically to ascertain the need for endodontic treatment
    E. Replant the tooth and advise him to see his dentist for endodontic treatment at 14–21 days

9. **A 56-year-old man undergoes a buccal advancement flap repair for an oro-antral fistula following removal of an upper first molar tooth. A few months later he returns with recurrent symptoms of a patent oro-antral communication coupled with ipsilateral sinus pain and evidence of mucosa thickening on computed tomography (CT) scanning. What is the next most appropriate step in management?**
    A. Repeat attempt at buccal advancement flap repair
    B. Buccal mucosal advancement flap with buccal fat pad (BFP) repair
    C. Buccal mucosal advancement flap with autogenous bone graft
    D. Palatal finger flap based on greater palatine artery
    E. Posterior pedicled inferior turbinate flap in combination with BFP and buccal mucosal advancement flap

10. **A 24-year-old woman with an impacted lower third molar deemed to be at high risk for an inferior alveolar nerve injury undergoes a coronectomy. Which of the following procedural errors is most likely to be related to the need for re-operation?**
    A. Failure to remove sufficient bone buccally
    B. Failure to mobilize the roots sufficiently
    C. Failure to remove enamel adequately
    D. Failure to provide watertight closure of the mucoperiosteal flap
    E. Failure to use lingual retraction

11. **Which of the following is regarded as a contraindication to coronectomy of an impacted lower third molar?**
    A. Loss of the lingual cortex on CBCT
    B. Altered shape of the inferior alveolar canal
    C. Preserved vitality of the third molar in question
    D. Incipient caries in the occlusal surface
    E. Horizontal impaction

12. **A 35-year-old man presents for an extraction of a carious but asymptomatic upper left second molar (UL7) under local anaesthesia. Upon elevating the tooth there is a sudden 'crack' with 'en bloc' movement of the upper left second molar (UL7), fully erupted third molar (UL8), and maxillary tuberosity. What is the next step in management?**

A. Explain the findings intraoperatively and complete the removal of both teeth along with the tuberosity, ensuring a repair of any oro-antral communication

B. Stop the procedure and rebook for beyond 6 weeks for a repeat attempt

C. Splint the UL78 to the adjacent teeth rigidly and rebook for beyond 6 weeks for a repeat attempt using a transalveolar (surgical) approach

D. Complete the procedure with a transalveolar (surgical) removal of the UL7, splinting the UL8 following completion

E. Remove the UL78 teeth and tuberosity but then separate the tuberosity ex vivo and replant this as a free bone graft prior to soft tissue closure

13. **Which of the following would *not* be regarded as indicative of an increased likelihood of maxillary tuberosity fracture during removal of an upper molar tooth?**

A. Enlarged maxillary sinus

B. Convergent root pattern

C. Lone standing maxillary molar tooth

D. Unerupted impacted third molar lying apical and distal to second molar

E. Hypercementosis

14. **A 16-year-old boy has an absent central incisor as a result of a traumatic injury and requires premolar extractions to facilitate fixed appliance orthodontic therapy. A treatment plan is proposed of autotransplantation of a premolar to the central incisor space. His parents ask what the likely success rate of this would be in terms of survival of the autotransplanted tooth. What is your response?**

A. 90% or greater

B. 70–90%

C. 50–70%

D. 30–50%

E. Less than 30%

15. **Which of the following features would be most likely to suggest that a patient should undergo exposure of an ectopic palatal canine rather than removal?**

A. Root resorption of the lateral incisor

B. Horizontal angulation

C. Close proximity of the canine to the midline

D. Good interproximal contact between the ipsilateral lateral incisor and first premolar teeth

E. A well-preserved retained deciduous canine

16. **A 47-year-old woman suffers hypoaesthesia affecting the sensory distribution of the right inferior alveolar nerve following removal of the right lower third molar. An agreement is reached with the patient to monitor for spontaneous recovery. Which size of Semmes–Weinstein filament is recommended for monitoring light touch?**

    A. 0.07 g
    B. 0.4 g
    C. 2.0 g
    D. 4.0 g
    E. 300 g

17. **Which of the following radiographic signs is *not* considered to be significant in predicting the likelihood of an injury to the inferior alveolar nerve during third molar surgery?**

    A. Radiolucency across the roots of the third molar
    B. Deviation of the mandibular canal
    C. Narrowing of the mandibular canal
    D. Deflection of the third molar roots by the canal
    E. Narrowing of the third molar root

18. **A patient sustains a Sunderland grade IV injury of the lingual nerve following removal of a third molar. What would be the most accurate description of this injury?**

    A. Neuropraxia or compression-type injury
    B. Neurotmesis
    C. Axonotmesis
    D. Lost axonal continuity with preservation of the endoneurium
    E. Lost axonal continuity with disrupted epineurium

19. **The asymptomatic patient in Figure 12.1 underwent an OPG radiograph as a new patient. Part of the radiograph is shown below. Which is the most appropriate next management?**

    A. Serial observation
    B. CT scan
    C. Reroot canal treatment of the lower premolar tooth
    D. Extraction of the first molar tooth
    E. Enucleation of the lesion

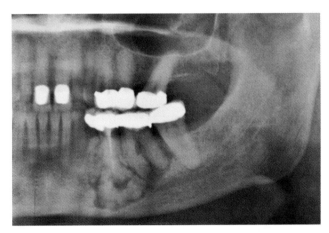

Figure 12.1 Part of an OPG radiograph showing a suspicious area in the mandible.

20. Which of the following is true of persistent idiopathic facial pain (PIFP)?

A. It has similar characteristics to trigeminal neuralgia

B. It should be distinguished from atypical facial pain

C. It has a relapsing, remitting quality

D. It has poor response to attempted treatments

E. It may demonstrate underlying pathology on T2-weighted magnetic resonance imaging (MRI)

21. Which of the following is correct regarding the area of fat that may be utilized in the procedure previously performed in Figure 12.2?

A. A fat only flap was previously undertaken

B. Infection due to fat necrosis has occurred

C. Fat pad perforation may have occurred

D. The fat pad is found superficial to the parotid duct

E. Excess fat harvesting may result in more pronounced jowls

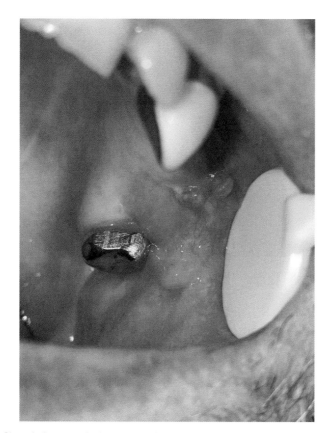

Figure 12.2 Clinical photograph showing an abnormality in the left buccal mucosa.

22. **The patient in Figure 12.3 presents with a skin abscess unresponsive to multiple courses of antibiotics. Pathology demonstrates granulomatous infection and Gram-positive bacteria with long-branching filaments but is otherwise non-diagnostic. Which of the following is true?**

    A. Mucosal trauma must have occurred
    B. Cervical lymphadenopathy would be expected
    C. Infection spreads along fascial planes
    D. Most patients will be immunocompromised
    E. Infection is due to acid fast bacilli

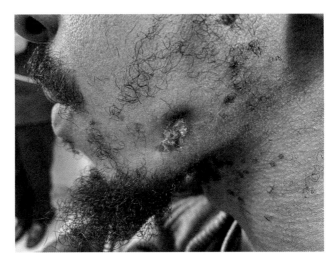

Figure 12.3 Clinical photograph showing an inflammatory area in the left cheek skin.

23. **The 28-year-old patient shown in the radiograph (Figure 12.4) has had two previous episodes of pericoronitis. Which of the following options represents the most appropriate management plan?**

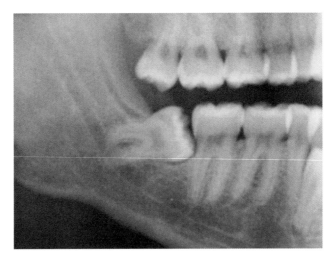

Figure 12.4 Part of an OPG radiograph showing a partially erupted mandibular third molar tooth.

    A. Conservative management with antibiotics when required
    B. Coronectomy
    C. Buccal bone removal then decoronation followed by root elevation
    D. Buccal bone removal then hemisection
    E. Sagittal split osteotomy

24. A 13-year-old patient has been referred to you for exposure and bonding of the canine tooth. Which of the following variables for canine position is not related to the favourability of this technique?

A. Rotation of canine crown in the horizontal plane

B. Vertical height of canine crown related to incisor

C. Angulation of canine to midline

D. Position of canine apex in the horizontal plane

E. Amount of canine horizontal overlap to incisor

25. An 11-year-old child sustains direct trauma to her maxillary teeth. Which of the following teeth is most likely to undergo necrosis?

A. Laterally luxated central incisor

B. Extruded first premolar

C. Intruded canine

D. Avulsed lateral incisor

E. Subluxated second premolar

1. A. Removal of the right third molar. There are relative contraindications to coronectomy, the appearances of the relationship with the nerve notwithstanding. The paper by Renton (2017) is a useful summary of the evidence base, but horizontal impaction and immunosuppression both weigh against the idea of a coronectomy. The paper by Omran et al. (2020) is a good overview of the position taken by Members and Fellows of the British Association of Oral and Maxillofacial Surgeons with regards to the place of coronectomy in practice. As the decision is tipped in favour of extraction rather than coronectomy, CBCT would arguably add little additional clinical information. There is no evidence that CBCT per se reduces the risk of nerve injury; rather it informs the discussion regarding a coronectomy, which is off the table here due to the nature of the impaction and the immunosuppression. Clearly these are relative contraindications and a discussion would still need to be had with the patient.

2. D. Mineral trioxide aggregate (MTA). Guidelines from the Royal College of Surgeons of England published in 2020 concerning periradicular surgery would suggest the use of MTA where moisture control proves difficult.

3. C. Surgical cricothyroidotomy. Guidelines described in the Difficult Airway Society are clear in a 'can't intubate, can't ventilate' situation that every measure should be tried first, such as head extension, jaw thrusts, and oral/nasal airway adjuncts. An LMA™, with maximum two attempts permitted, comes next. The key here is that a person trained in advanced airway skills has tried to intubate the patient via the standard approach and failed. A surgical cricothyroidotomy would balance efficiency and speed with the ability to effectively ventilate the patient rather than merely insufflate.

4. D. Lingual retraction with a purpose-built retractor. The evidence base for and against lingual retraction in third molar surgery is heterogenous, with arguments cited for and against (and medicolegal cases settled either way!). A recent systematic review published by Rapaport and Brown (2020) highlighted that whilst no lingual retraction and repurposed retractors showed tangible rates of permanent injury to the lingual nerve (0.08% and 0.41%, respectively), the use of purpose-built retractors was the only method related to a 0% incidence of permanent injury.

5. C. Within 3 months. The success of exploratory surgery for iatrogenic injuries of the inferior alveolar and lingual nerves has been related to the time from injury to repair in a number of studies. It is generally a consensus view that if spontaneous recovery is not forthcoming by 90 days, a referral should occur, with the aim of surgery happening at 3–6 months post injury. This is explained well in a systematic review by Kushnerev and Yates (2015).

6. A. Cognitive behavioural therapy (CBT). In iatrogenic trigeminal nerve injuries, the success of surgery is consistently related to the time from the initial injury to exploration and repair. Topical and systemic medications really only have a role in the management of neuropathic pain. Many patients with hypoaesthesia or anaesthesia alone in a series by Renton et al in 2012 responded well to reassurance and counselling alone, but a small proportion (8%) required CBT.

7. E. Superior cluneal nerve. All the other nerves are at risk except the superior cluneal nerve, which relates only to posterior iliac crest harvest.

8. C. Replant the tooth and splint with a flexible splint for up to 14 days. The Dental Trauma Guide available online is an excellent resource concerning the management of traumatic injuries to the permanent and primary dentition. The advice for an avulsed closed apex tooth with an extra-alveolar dry time of greater than 60 minutes includes flexible splinting for less than 14 days. Endodontic treatment is essential and the time to extirpation has been shown to relate to success rates and the incidence of replacement resorption.

9. E. Posterior pedicled inferior turbinate flap in combination with BFP and buccal mucosal advancement flap. The three-layered technique described by Darr et al. (2018) enables a more robust closure (albeit necessitating general anaesthesia) and enables simultaneous treatment of the co-existing sinus disease, which may have contributed to the failure here. The stress in the question is the sinus changes. He would benefit from an antrostomy and washout arguably, and he has had a failed standard approach.

10. C. Failure to remove enamel adequately. Inadequate enamel removal has been shown to relate most strongly to the need for re-operation following coronectomy in a number of studies to date, as demonstrated in a histopathological study of retained roots published by Patel et al. (2014).

11. E. Horizontal impaction. Horizontal impaction is as a relative contraindication due to difficulty in obtaining a successful coronectomy as a result of the high placement of the retained root surface in relation to the alveolus.

12. C. Splint the UL78 to the adjacent teeth rigidly and rebook for beyond 6 weeks for a repeat attempt using a transalveolar (surgical) approach . There is little in the way of consensus opinion here, with advice being given on a case-by-case basis. Ultimately, were the tooth to be infected or symptomatic, every effort should be made to complete the procedure. Given that it is asymptomatic, it would be reasonable to allow bony healing and then perform an elective surgical approach at a later date to optimize chances of preserving the tuberosity and the UL8. In the case of smaller tuberosity fractures, the lesser of two evils may be to remove the fragment of bone along with the tooth (e.g. the case of a last standing tooth).

13. B. Convergent root pattern. All the other answers are risk factors except for convergent root pattern, as divergent roots are regarded as an additional risk factor. Other risk factors include reduced thickness of the buccal plate, mesiodistal space loss in the case of grossly carious teeth, a low-lying antral floor in between the teeth, heavily restored teeth, fused teeth (concrescence), and multirooted teeth.

14. A. 90% or greater. Whilst early attempts at autotransplantation yielded success rates of around 50%, the largest series published by Andreasen et al. in 1990 of 370 transplanted premolar teeth demonstrated that 86% exhibited normal healing, 13.9% were clinically successful (but showed radiographic evidence of root resorption), and only 0.1% required extraction. Other, albeit smaller series, have shown similar outcomes, with success enhanced by conical root morphology, immature teeth, surgical skill, and multidisciplinary team planning.

15.   A. Root resorption of the lateral incisor. Guidelines on the management of ectopic canines are available from the Faculty of Dental Surgery of the Royal College of Surgeons of England in 2016. Root resorption of the lateral incisor would steer the treatment plan towards removing the compromised tooth and aligning the retained canine in its stead.

16.   C. 2.0 g. Whilst light touch can be monitored simply using a cotton bud or similar, reproducibility is better achieved with a standardized technique such as Semmes–Weinstein filaments or von Frey hairs. A 20-mN or 2.0-g filament is recommended for this sensory area. We have included this question purposefully, as medicolegally this is the standard used by UK hospital units with a focus on nerve repair, like Sheffield.

17.   C. Narrowing of the mandibular canal. Whilst few studies have been done on this matter, the seminal work by Rood and Shehab (1990) is regarded as the basis for much work that followed on this subject. Certainly, the radiographic signs they identified should prompt strong consideration of CBCT scans and the offer of a coronectomy.

18.   C. Axonotmesis. There are two classification schema used to describe nerve injuries. The first was published by Seddon in 1943, and separated injuries into three categories — neuropraxia, axonotmesis, and neurotmesis — largely based on the scale of injury from microscopic to macroscopic. In 1978, Sunderland expanded upon this idea, subdividing neurotmesis into three additional grades. The Seddon classification is useful to understand the anatomic basis for injury, while the Sunderland classification adds information useful for prognosis and treatment strategies. A Sunderland grade IV injury includes endoneurial and perineurial injury along with transection of the axon, but preservation of the epineurium. It is a subclassification of an axonotmesis-type injury.

19.   A. Serial observation. This patient has an area of fibro-osseous dysplasia. Without looking at the complete radiograph it is not possible to tell if it is just focal and not florid, but an additional CT scan is not required. The radiolucency around the first molar tooth is likely an early part of the whole lesion. The reroot treatment, although of dubious quality, was likely a misdiagnosis of another early lesion.

20.   D. It has poor response to attempted treatments. Recently the term persistent idiopathic facial pain (PIFP) has widely replaced atypical facial pain. In the 2nd Edition of the International Classification of Headache Disorders, PIFP is defined as 'persistent facial pain that does not have the characteristics of the cranial neuralgias and is not attributed to another disorder'. There are no objective examination findings or test results, no obvious explanation for the cause of the pain, and a poor response to attempted treatments.

21.   C. Fat pad perforation may have occurred. The clinical photograph demonstrates a buccal advancement flap as evidenced by loss of vestibule. Intraoperative BFP perforation is an indication for two-layer closure. The anterior lobe of the BFP encapsulates the parotid duct. There is evidence of persistent infection, which is most likely due to chronic sinusitis. The mean volume of the BFP is 10 ml, and excess harvesting may depress the cheek and may accentuate the nasolabial fold.

22.   A. Mucosal trauma must have occurred. This patient has cervicofacial actinomycosis, an infection characterized by granulomatous and suppurative lesions. Cervical lymphadenopathy is a late presentation. Although bacterial culture of the oral commensal Actinomycetaceae is the gold standard for definitive diagnosis, this can be highly challenging to achieve. Bacilli are not acid fast. Mucosal trauma is the primary causative mechanism, and although actinomycosis affects immunocompromised people, most reported cases have been in immunocompetent people.

23. A. Conservative management with antibiotics when required. This radiograph demonstrates a bifid mandibular canal, a variant of normal. Anatomical studies have shown that the upper canal with this particular appearance is likely to traverse the tooth itself or run immediately buccally to the tooth. Damage to this top branch may still cause altered sensation despite the presence of the lower branch. It may also result in neuroma formation and an increased risk of bleeding.

24. A. Rotation of canine crown in the horizontal plane. This is false. The other answers are the four aspects of canine position that should be assessed, as well as the patient's age, as described by McSherry et al.

25. A. Laterally luxated central incisor. Whether pulp necrosis will occur following trauma depends on the type of injury and stage of root development. The risk of pulp necrosis is least after concussion and subluxation and greatest in extrusion, lateral luxation, and intrusion, in that order. In immature teeth with an open apex, revascularization following luxation or avulsion may occur. The apex of a lateral incisor closes at approximately 11 years old.

References

Andreasen JO, Paulsen HU, Yu Z, Ahlquist R, Bayer T, Schwartz O (1990). A long-term study of 370 autotransplanted premolars. Part I. Surgical procedures and standardized techniques for monitoring healing. *European Journal of Orthodontics* **12**(1):3–13. doi:10.1093/ejo/12.1.3. PMID: 2318261.

Darr A, Jolly K, Martin T, Monaghan A, Grime P, Isles M, Beech T, Ahmed S (2018). Three-layered technique to repair an oroantral fistula using a posterior-pedicled inferior turbinate, buccal fat pad, and buccal mucosal advancement flap. *British Journal of Oral and Maxillofacial Surgery* **56**(7):638–639.

Dental Trauma Guide. Available at: https://dentaltraumaguide.org

Frerk C, Mitchell VS, McNarry AF, Mendonca C, Bhagrath R, Patel A, O'Sullivan EP, Woodall NM, Ahmad I (2015). Difficult Airway Society intubation guidelines working group. Difficult Airway Society 2015 guidelines for management of unanticipated difficult intubation in adults. *British Journal of Anaesthesia* **115**(6):827–848.

Headache Classification Committee of The International Headache Society. The International Classification of Headache Disorders (second edition). Available at: http://216.25.100.131/ihscommon/guidelines/pdfs/ihc_II_main_no_print.pdf

Husain J, Burden D, McSherry P (2016). Guidelines on the management of ectopic canines. Faculty of Dental Surgery. Royal College of Surgeons of England. Available at: https://www.rcseng.ac.uk/dental-faculties/fds/publications-guidelines/clinical-guidelines/

Kushnerev E, Yates JM (2015). Evidence-based outcomes following inferior alveolar and lingual nerve injury and repair: a systematic review. *Journal of Oral Rehabilitation* **42**(10):786–802.

McSherry PF (1998). The ectopic maxillary canine: a review. *British Journal of Orthodontics* **25**(3):209–216.

Omran A, Hutchison I, Ridout F, Bose A, Maroni R, Dhanda J, Hammond D, Moynihan C, Ciniglio A, Chiu G (2020). Current perspectives on the surgical management of mandibular third molars in the United Kingdom: the need for further research. *British Journal of Oral and Maxillofacial Surgery* **58**(3):348–354.

Patel V, Sproat C, Kwok J, Beneng K, Thavaraj S, McGurk M (2014). Histological evaluation of mandibular third molar roots retrieved after coronectomy. *British Journal of Oral and Maxillofacial Surgery* **52**(5):415–419.

Rapaport BHJ, Brown JS (2020). Systematic review of lingual nerve retraction during surgical mandibular third molar extractions. *British Journal of Oral and Maxillofacial Surgery* **58**(7):748–752.

Renton T (2017). Risk assessment of M3Ms and decisions on ordering a CBCT and prescribing a coronectomy. *Dental Update* **44**(10):957–976.

Renton T, Yilmaz Z, Gaballah K (2012). Evaluation of trigeminal nerve injuries in relation to third molar surgery in a prospective patient cohort. Recommendations for prevention. *International Journal of Oral and Maxillofacial Surgery* **41**(12):1509–1518.

Renton T, Yilmaz Z (2012). Managing iatrogenic trigeminal nerve injury: a case series and review of the literature. *International Journal of Oral and Maxillofacial Surgery* **41**(5):629–637.

Rood JP, Shehab BA (1990). The radiological prediction of inferior alveolar nerve injury during third molar surgery. *British Journal of Oral and Maxillofacial Surgery* **28**(1):20–25.

Royal College of Surgeons of England (2020). Guidelines for periradicular Surgery. London: RCS England. Available at: https://www.rcseng.ac.uk/dental-faculties/fds/publications-guidelines/clinical-guidelines/

Seddon HJ (1943). Peripheral Nerve Injuries. *Glasgow Medical Journal* **139**(3):61–75.

Sunderland S (1951). A classification of peripheral nerve injuries producing loss of function. *Brain* **74**(4):491–516. doi:10.1093/brain/74.4.491. PMID: 14895767.

1. **Which of the following is true of the temporoparietal fascia flap?**
    A. It becomes the parotid-masseteric fascia inferiorly
    B. It can be utilized as a sensory flap
    C. Skin and cartilage can be incorporated from the helical rim
    D. The blood supply is from the occipital and superficial temporal artery and venae
    E. It has an 8-cm-long pedicle enabling versatility

2. **A 48-year-old man who smokes heavily develops osteomyelitis resulting in a pathological fracture of his right mandible. Following resolution with removal of a causative first molar, debridement, and 6 weeks of intravenous antibiotics in the community, he shows complete resolution of the osteomyelitis at 3 months but a segmental mandibular defect of around 5 cm with complete mucosal coverage. What is the reconstructive method of choice?**
    A. Iliac crest free corticocancellous graft
    B. Distal circumflex iliac artery (DCIA) flap
    C. Fibula flap
    D. Scapula flap
    E. Pectoralis major myocutaneous (PMMC) flap

3. **Which of the following flaps is a perforator-based chimeric flap?**
    A. Fibula flap with skin paddle
    B. Anterolateral thigh flap with two skin paddles
    C. Scapula flap
    D. Composite radial forearm flap
    E. PMMC flap

4. **A latissimus dorsi flap is what type of flap according to the Mathes and Nahai classification of muscular flaps?**
    A. Type I
    B. Type II
    C. Type III
    D. Type IV
    E. Type V

5. A 54-year-old man undergoes a partial maxillectomy encompassing the orbital floor, although the orbital contents are retained. He is keen to have fixed prosthodontic rehabilitation as soon as feasible following his surgery. Which reconstructive option would be the optimal choice for this patient?
    A. Non-vascularized iliac crest
    B. DCIA flap
    C. Composite radial forearm free flap
    D. Osteocutaneous scapula flap
    E. Vascularized fibula flap

6. A patient undergoes a deltopectoral island flap for reconstruction of a cutaneous defect low down in the anterior neck. What is the dominant blood supply?
    A. Clavicular branch of the thoracoacromial artery
    B. Pectoral branch of the thoracoacromial artery
    C. Pectoral branch of the lateral thoracic artery
    D. Perforating branches of the internal mammary artery
    E. Perforating branches of the intercostal arteries

7. During a fibula flap harvest the pedicle of the peroneal artery and veins is exposed through dividing the chevron-shaped fibres of which muscle?
    A. Peroneus longus
    B. Peroneus brevis
    C. Extensor hallucis longus
    D. Tibialis anterior
    E. Tibialis posterior

8. Following a fibula flap harvest, a 56-year-old woman begins physiotherapy but it is noted that she is unable to evert her foot and has lost some sensation over the dorsum of her foot. Which nerve is likely to have been injured?
    A. Lateral sural cutaneous nerve
    B. Deep peroneal nerve
    C. Common peroneal nerve
    D. Superficial peroneal nerve
    E. Intermediate dorsal cutaneous nerve

9. **Which of the following statements is true concerning scapular flaps?**

    A. The scapular flap skin paddle is supplied by the vertical (descending) branch of the circumflex scapular artery

    B. The circumflex scapular artery may originate directly from the axillary artery

    C. The blood supply of the medial border of the scapula comes from the superficial branch of the dorsal scapular artery

    D. The superficial cutaneous branch of the circumflex scapular artery passes through the quadrangular space

    E. The triangular space is bounded by the humerus laterally and the teres minor and teres major muscles

10. **A 56-year-old man has undergone reconstruction of a segmental defect in his mandible with a vascularized free fibula flap. No skin paddle was required for the flap. On the fifth day post-operatively he exhibits an intermittent fever, white cell count of $18.1 \times 10^9/l$, and C-reactive protein of 134 mg/l. Urinalysis and a plain film chest radiograph are both normal. What additional investigation would be most useful?**

    A. Plain film radiograph of the mandible

    B. Duplex sonography

    C. Computed tomography (CT) scan of the neck with contrast

    D. Technetium-99m (99mTc)-methylene diphosphonate scan

    E. Fluorodeoxyglucose (FDG) positron emission tomography (PET) scan

11. **A 38-year-old woman sustained injury to the buccal and zygomatic branches following removal of a benign tumour from the right parotid gland some 20 months prior to her attendance in your clinic. She is most concerned about asymmetry of her smile. Which of the following options would provide her with a spontaneous smile?**

    A. Tensor fasciae latae sling

    B. Cross-facial nerve graft

    C. Interpositional nerve graft with the sural nerve

    D. Free gracilis muscle transfer utilizing the masseteric nerve

    E. Free gracilis muscle transfer utilizing the cross-facial nerve graft

12. **With regards to posterior cranial vault remodeling, which of the following is true?**

    A. The patient is placed supine with the head secured in a three-pin headrest

    B. Exposure of the skull posteriorly is required past the lambdoid suture

    C. Craniotomy enables a bandeau segment to be discarded

    D. Barrel stave osteotomies allow for expansive cranial width correction

    E. Bicortical bone grafts are harvested from the osteotomized segments

13. **Which of the following regarding Figure 13.1 are true?**

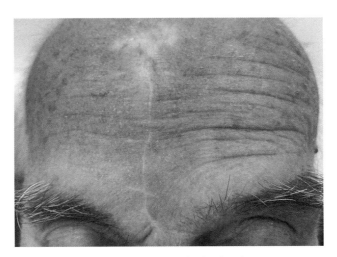

Figure 13.1 Clinical photograph showing a scar on the forehead.

A. Subperiosteal dissection should start just above the supraorbital rim
B. Extending the flap at right angles to increase pedicle length is contraindicated
C. The vascular bundle lies 1.2–1.7 cm lateral to the midline
D. The artery remains submuscular until approximately 1.0 cm above the foramen
E. The recipient site is likely to be contralateral

14. **Which is the most appropriate flap to repair a 9-cm-diameter multicystic ameloblastoma affecting the angle of the mandible? The patient has a history of a proximal fibular fracture**

A. Fibular free flap
B. Non-vascularized iliac crest graft
C. Deep circumflex iliac artery flap
D. Radial forearm flap
E. Scapular free flap

15. **Methods to optimize monitoring of microvascular free flaps include all but which one of the following?**

A. If the haematocrit falls below 0.25 a blood transfusion should be considered
B. Near infrared spectroscopy is superior to laser Doppler
C. Temperature difference greater than 2°C between the flap and the core signifies possible flap ischaemia
D. Reduced haemoglobin oxygenation detected by pulse oximetry may signify increased risk of failure
E. If the haematocrit rises above 0.35 colloid should be given

1. **C. Skin and cartilage can be incorporated from the helical rim.** The temporoparietal fascia is an extension of the subcutaneous musculoaponeurotic system (SMAS) inferiorly and the galea aponeurotica superiorly. The blood supply is from the posterior branches from the superficial temporal artery and venae. The superficial temporal artery is small calibre, with a short pedicle of up to 3 cm long at best.

2. **A. Iliac crest free corticocancellous graft.** Pogrel's 1997 paper on comparisons between vascularized and non-vascularized grafts for mandibular continuity defects highlighted the latter being comparable for defects less than 9 cm in length. This figure has been reduced to possibly 6 cm by other authorities (including the Birmingham group, Nandra et al. 2017), but ultimately short spans with complete mucosal coverage would lend themselves to simpler reconstructive options, with the caveat that implant survival is not as predictable.

3. **B. Anterolateral thigh flap with two skin paddles.** A chimeric flap is defined as one with independent flaps with independent vascular supply emanating from a common source vessel. Huang et al. (2003) have subdivided these based on specific blood supply, with a multiple paddle anterolateral thigh flap epitomizing a perforator-based chimeric flap, lending itself to relining intraoral and extraoral defects simultaneously.

4. **E. Type V.** Mathes and Nahai published a classification system of muscular flaps in 1981 and it remains a useful classification system. The type V is a flap based on a single dominant pedicle and multiple secondary segmental vessels. Its dominant supply stems from the thoracodorsal artery (a branch of the subscapular artery), with the secondary supply originating from posterior intercostal perforators.

5. **B. Deep circumflex iliac artery (DCIA) flap.** This is a Brown class III maxillectomy defect, and whilst fibula flaps are an option, the DCIA is the preferred reconstruction, as explained in Brown and Shaw (2010). Vascularized flaps are vastly superior in terms of supporting implant-retained prosthodontics, with the iliac crest being demonstrated as the most consistently implantable donor site in a series published by Moscoso et al. (1994).

6. **D. Perforating branches of the internal mammary artery.** The deltopectoral flap is not commonly utilized and is often viewed as a 'back-up to the back-up' option that the PMMC flap has become. The dominant blood supply is the second or third perforating branches of the internal mammary artery. For this reason, one may think twice about using this in someone with ischaemic heart disease who may later need their internal mammary artery for a coronary artery bypass!

7. **E. Tibialis posterior.** The characteristic shape and direction of the fibres are a good clue to when one is approaching the pedicle for this flap and to avoiding confusion with the anterior tibial vessels.

8. **D. Superficial peroneal nerve.**   This nerve is a branch of the common peroneal nerve, which supplies motor function specifically to the peroneus longus and peroneus brevis muscles and sensory supply to the skin over the lower one-third of the lateral side of the leg and much of the dorsum of the foot. It is prone to neuropraxia during harvest of the fibula flap.

9. **B. The circumflex scapular artery may originate directly from the axillary artery.** Whilst the circumflex scapular artery most commonly originates from the inferior scapular, a direct origin from the axillary artery may be the case in around 3% of instances.

10. **C. Computed tomography (CT) scan of the neck with contrast.**   In this clinical scenario the change in clinical parameters at day five would suggest a collection of pus such as an infected haematoma, although the non-viability of the flap must be borne in mind. A CT scan would show a collection of pus, haematoma, or fat necrosis from dead bone and thereby ascertain if drainage was required. A non-viable flap can potentially be detected with a 99mTc-methylene diphosphonate scan, but in most hospitals such a scan cannot be done acutely. The absence of the skin paddle means clinical monitoring is impossible, although continuous monitoring methods have now come to the fore in modern practice (e.g. Cook–Swartz implantable Doppler probes).

11. **E. Free gracilis muscle transfer utilizing the cross-facial nerve graft.**   Given the time that has elapsed, cross-facial nerve grafts alone are not an option, as the muscle will have atrophied. A dynamic repair is warranted and spontaneity can only really be established utilizing the natural nerve supply for facial expression, as using the masseteric would instead be 'learned'.

12. **D. Barrel stave osteotomies allow for expansive cranial width correction.**   The patient is placed prone with the head secured in a padded Mayfield horseshoe headrest. A bicoronal incision is made to expose the skull posteriorly past the superior nuchal line. Craniotomy enables skull segments to be osteotomized and a bandeau harvested. Barrel stave osteotomies allow for expansive cranial width correction. Bone grafts are harvested from the inner table of the osteotomized segments.

13. **D. The artery remains submuscular until approximately 1.0 cm above the foramen.**   Maintaining an axial pattern, utilizing the pedicle ipsilateral to the defect, extending the flap at right angles with caution when extra length is needed, using a narrow pedicle, and early subperiosteal dissection are the guiding principles of the paramedian flap. The anatomic studies of Shumrick and Smith demonstrate the position and course of the supratrochlear artery, running 1.7–2.2 cm lateral to the midline in a vertical vector. The artery runs in the submuscular plane to a more superficial, subcutaneous position beginning 1 cm above the brow.

14. **A. Fibular free flap.**   The size of this defect practically precludes harvest of any free flap other than a fibula. Many surgeons would often be hesitant in its use in patients with a history of distal fibular fracture, but less with a proximal fracture. The lateral aspect of the scapula can be harvested to a size of 1–2 cm wide and up to 10 cm long. The radial forearm flap can provide thin, pliable skin and a maximum of 10 cm of bone, which can include a cross-sectional area comprising approximately 40% of the radius.

15. **D. Reduced haemoglobin oxygenation detected by pulse oximetry may signify increased risk of failure.**   This is incorrect. The haematocrit should be maintained between 0.25 and 0.35 in adults. If it falls below 0.25 blood transfusion should be considered. If it rises above 0.35 colloid should be given. Near-infrared spectroscopy is similar to laser Doppler but utilizes a longer wavelength of light and consequently penetrates deeper. Pulse oximetry is useful for monitoring digital replants but has limited value for flaps to the head and neck region.

References

Brown JS, Shaw RJ (2010). Reconstruction of the maxilla and midface: introducing a new classification. *Lancet Oncology* **11**(10):1001–1008.

Huang WC, Chen HC, Wei FC, Cheng MH, Schnur DP (2003). Chimeric flap in clinical use. *Clinics in Plastic Surgery* **30**(3):457–467.

Mathes SJ, Nahai F (1981). Classification of the vascular anatomy of muscles: experimental and clinical correlation. *Plastic and Reconstructive Surgery* **67**(2):177–187.

Moscoso JF, Urken ML (1994). The iliac crest composite flap for oromandibular reconstruction. *Otolaryngologic Clinics of North America* **27**(6):1097–117.

Nandra B, Fattahi T, Martin T, Praveen P, Fernandes R, Parmar S (2017). Free Bone Grafts for Mandibular Reconstruction in Patients Who Have Not Received Radiotherapy: The 6-cm Rule-Myth or Reality? *Craniomaxillofacial Trauma & Reconstruction* **10**(2):117–122.

Pogrel MA, Podlesh S, Anthony JP, Alexander J (1997). A comparison of vascularized and nonvascularized bone grafts for reconstruction of mandibular continuity defects. *Journal of Oral and Maxillofacial Surgery* **55**(11):1200–1206.

Shumrick KA, Smith TL (1992). The anatomic basis for the design of forehead flaps in nasal reconstruction. *Archives of Otorhinolaryngology-Head & Neck Surgery* **118**(4):373–379.

1. Which of the following statements about bone density is true?

A. D2 bone is found in the posterior maxilla
B. Sinus grafting generally results in D3 bone
C. There is a direct correlation between bone density and implant survival
D. Bone quality can be determined from Hounsfield units (HU)
E. Dense cortical bone equates to HU <1,000

2. You review an implant that you placed in the anterior maxilla 6 months ago. The patient is asymptomatic, but probing around the implant reaches a 7-mm depth but the gingiva appears healthy. There are no radiographic changes. What does this most likely represent?

A. Normal functioning
B. Peri-implantitis
C. Implant failure
D. Component failure
E. Parafunction

3. The future height of interdental papillae in the aesthetic zone of a single missing tooth is affected by which one of the following?

A. Interproximal bone height of the adjacent teeth
B. Gingival biotype
C. Flap design
D. Provisional crown shape
E. All of the above

4. When selecting an osteointegrated dental implant, which of the following is true?

A. It is best to choose the longest implant possible, because the longest implants survive best
B. It is best to choose the widest implant possible, because the widest implants survive best
C. Implant surface selection is critical
D. At least 1 mm of bone lingual and buccal of the implant must remain for it to survive
E. Implants are contraindicated in patients taking some antidepressants and antithrombotic agents

5. **A failing dental implant shows an increase in which groups of subgingival microorganisms?**
   A. *Streptococcus mutans*
   B. Aerobic Gram-negative bacteria
   C. Anaerobic Gram-negative bacteria
   D. Black-pigmented *Porphyromonas*
   E. Anaerobic Gram-positive bacteria

6. **Which of the following statements is false about antibiotic prophylaxis in clean contaminated maxillofacial surgical procedures?**
   A. Antibiotic prophylaxis is not routinely indicated for lower third molar surgery
   B. Antibiotic prophylaxis is not routinely indicated for placing a routine dental implant
   C. Antibiotic prophylaxis is indicated for minor surgery with a high degree of difficulty in which the duration of the surgery is predicted to be long
   D. Antibiotic prophylaxis is indicated for open reduction and internal fixation of midface bone fractures
   E. Antibiotics are not indicated post-operatively following open reduction and internal fixation of the mandible

7. **Which of the following is true for the concept of All-on-4® dental implants?**
   A. It can refer to either fixed or removable prostheses
   B. The prosthesis is fitted up to 1 week following fixture placement
   C. The posterior implants are placed at an angle
   D. It necessitates pre-operative cone beam computed tomography (CBCT) imaging
   E. It can be utilized in partially dentate patients

8. **The patient with the radiograph shown in Figure 14.1 attends with recurrent facial swelling resistant to two courses of co-amoxiclav. They had teeth extracted 3 months ago in preparation for All-On-4® dental implants. Which of the following is the most appropriate next course of management?**
   A. CBCT
   B. Biopsy
   C. Caldwell–Luc surgical access
   D. Endoscopic sinus retrieval
   E. Low-dose clindamycin

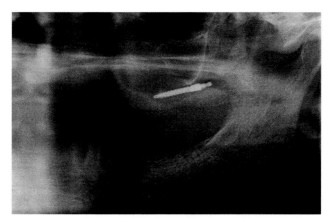

Figure 14.1 Radiopacity noted incidentally on an OPG radiograph.

9. **Which of the following is true of the method of implant prosthesis attachment shown in Figure 14.2 compared to using a screw?**

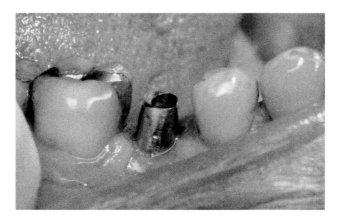

Figure 14.2 Clinical radiograph of part of a dental implant.

A. It is more aesthetic
B. It is harder to place when mouth opening is limited
C. It is harder to fabricate
D. It has more complications
E. It requires less abutment height

10. A patient with the radiograph shown in Figure 14.3 attends with pain around their implant retained crown 6 months after placement. Examination demonstrates erythema around the prosthesis but no increased pocketing. What does this most likely represent?

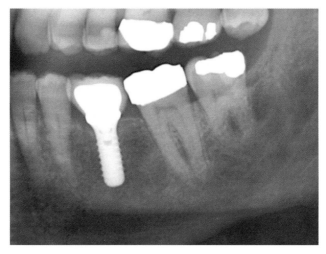

Figure 14.3 Part of an OPG radiograph showing a dental implant.

    A. Implant failure
    B. Peri-implantitis
    C. Fracture of a component
    D. Loosening of a component
    E. Occlusal parafunction

1. B. Sinus grafting generally results in D3 bone. This, however, will not occur until approximately 6 months after grafting. Bone density is classified by Misch into D1–D5. The posterior maxilla is D4 bone and is the least dense of the jaws. There is weak correlation between this classification and survival rates. HU are an indication only of bone density and not quality. Dense cortical bone is generally only found in the resorbed anterior mandible and has HU >1,250.

2. A. Normal functioning. This presentation would suggest normal functioning. Signs of inflammation are common with peri-implantitis. In addition, signs of inflammation and radiographic changes are likely with implant and component failures. Parafunction, predominantly bruxism, is generally considered a contraindication for implant treatment, although causational evidence between bruxism and failure is lacking.

3. E. All of the above. Incisions that spare at least 1 mm of the papilla are required to ensure that papilla necrosis does not occur. Mucoperiosteal flaps if raised should avoid the labial aspect. A thick biotype resists recession, is able to better conceal titanium, and helps maintain gingival morphology.

4. D. At least 1 mm of bone lingual and buccal of the implant must remain for it to survive. Survival rates are only compromised when implants are very short and bone density is poor. There is no such correlation of survival with width. Either smooth or rough surfaces can be used for implants, although rough surfaces seem preferable. A higher failure rate of implants placed in sites with history of implant failure occurs in patients taking antidepressants and antithrombotic agents, but they are not an absolute contraindication.

5. C. Anaerobic Gram-negative bacteria. Stable implants have microbiota similar to that found in healthy periodontium, predominantly Gram-positive anaerobic cocci and rods. In contrast, failing implants have bacteria similar to the ones seen in periodontal disease, including *Prevotella intermedia*, *Fusobacterium* spp., and spirochetes. These anaerobic Gram-negative bacilli are common elements of the mucous membrane flora throughout the body and often act as secondary pathogens.

6. B. Antibiotic prophylaxis is not routinely indicated for placing a routine dental implant. Grade A evidence based upon a Cochrane Review led by Esposito et al. demonstrates that antibiotic prophylaxis is indicated for surgery to place dental implants. There is grade B evidence that antibiotic prophylaxis is indicated for open reduction and internal fixation of facial bone fractures, but that it should not be continued post-operatively.

7. C. The posterior implants are placed at an angle. The All-On-4® technique is used to rehabilitate completely edentulous patients. Four implants support two fixed prostheses, each with 10–14 teeth. It is typically fitted within 24 hours of surgery. The two posterior implants are placed at an angle to avoid the maxillary sinus and inferior alveolar nerve canal. Although CBCT imaging continues to grow in popularity, it is not currently a prerequisite for this technique.

8. B. Biopsy. The implant in the sinus is a distraction and the focus should instead be on the radiolucency in the left mandible. The patient most likely has osteonecrosis of the mandible, although bone metastases from the breast, bronchus, kidney, prostate, and colon cannot be excluded. A biopsy is required to establish the diagnosis, followed by a conventional CT scan. The retained implant should be removed before another implant is placed. This would need to be through a Caldwell–Luc approach as the implant length would preclude endoscopic retrieval.

9. A. It is more aesthetic. This image shows an abutment for a cemented dental implant prostheses. Compared to a screw-retained prosthesis, cemented prostheses are easier to fabricate, easier to attach when mouth opening is limited, generally have better aesthetics, and overall have fewer complications. They do, however, require an abutment height of at least 5 mm.

10. D. Loosening of a component. Clinical inflammation around a single restored implant, associated with pain, but no radiographic bone loss, is most likely due to component loosening. Component fracture would likely have led to the prosthesis detaching and peri-implantitis usually demonstrates radiologically visible bone loss.

Reference

Esposito M, Grusovin MG, Worthington HV (2013). Interventions for replacing missing teeth: antibiotics at dental implant placement to prevent complications. *Cochrane Database of Systematic Reviews* **2013**(7):CD004152.

1. **Following a dorsal hump reduction, failure to perform lateral osteotomies will lead to which deformity post rhinoplasty?**
   A. Pollybeak deformity
   B. Open roof deformity
   C. Inverted V deformity
   D. Rocker deformity
   E. Increased columella display

2. **Which of the following tip refinements can be made through a closed rhinoplasty approach?**
   A. Depressor septi nasi division
   B. Shield graft placement
   C. Transdomal suturing
   D. Interdomal suturing
   E. Cephalic trim of the lower lateral cartilages

3. **Which nerve is most commonly injured during a rhytidectomy?**
   A. Marginal mandibular nerve
   B. Greater auricular nerve
   C. Auriculotemporal nerve
   D. Frontal branch of the facial nerve
   E. Masseteric nerve

4. **As an adjunct to a minimal access cranial suspension (MACS) facelift, the surgeon decides to correct contour deficiencies as a result of some superficial static perioral rhytids with a technique that also achieves a rejuvenating effect in the skin. What technique is employed?**
   A. Coleman fat transfer
   B. Microfat grafting
   C. Nanofat grafting
   D. Hyaluronic acid filler
   E. Botulinum toxin injections

5. **Which of the following technique is not advisable in the treatment of established keloid scar formation?**

   A. Scar excision with Z-plasty for reorientation
   B. Intralesional triamcinolone acetonide
   C. Intralesional excision
   D. Electron beam radiation therapy
   E. Silicone sheeting

6. **Following a chemical peel with 20% trichloracetic acid, a 25-year-old woman develops a patchy vesicular rash. Which medication should have been prescribed peri procedure?**

   A. 0.05–0.1% all-trans retinoic acid
   B. Acyclovir
   C. Blue Peel®
   D. Prednisolone
   E. Ganciclovir

7. **A 91-year-old man with ischaemic heart disease and chronic obstructive pulmonary disease has a squamous cell carcinoma removed from his right temple. Histopathology confirms a moderately differentiated tumour, which has been removed with adequate margins and no adjuvant treatment is required. He has sustained frontal branch palsy, however, which is still present at 3 months. This interferes with his weekly game of snooker. What would be your recommended treatment?**

   A. Cross-facial nerve graft (CFNG)
   B. Botulinum toxin to the contralateral forehead
   C. Direct brow lift
   D. Endoscopic brow lift with Endotine®
   E. Tensor fascia lata (TFL) static sling

8. **Following a rhinoplasty, the patient complains of difficulty breathing, particularly during exertion. Examination reveals supra-alar pinching with external valve compromise. What corrective measure can be undertaken?**

   A. Alar batten grafts
   B. Shield graft
   C. Caudal extension graft
   D. Columellar strut graft
   E. Securing the medial crura to the caudal septum

9. **What is the ideal source of innervated muscle transfer for dynamic repair of a unilateral lower lip palsy?**
    A. Digastric
    B. Platysma
    C. Frontalis
    D. Gracilis
    E. Masseter

10. **A 56-year-old woman presents with mild (2–3 mm) mechanical ptosis due to dermatochalasis and excellent levator function. What technique would you use to correct this?**
    A. Kuhnt–Szymanowski procedure
    B. Fasanella–Servat tarso-mullerectomy
    C. External levator aponeurosis advancement
    D. Supra-Whitnall's ligament levator muscle resection
    E. Frontalis muscle suspension with autogenous fascia lata

11. **You are called to review a patient with facial fractures and burns who was involved in an explosion at the workplace. The patient can feel you gently touching their dark pink skin. The capillary refill time is approximately 3 seconds. What level of burn is this?**
    A. Superficial
    B. Superficial dermal
    C. Mid-dermal
    D. Deep dermal
    E. Full thickness

12. **You are about to perform a lower blepharoplasty. There is minimal lid skin laxity. Which of the following is not true regarding the fat pads?**
    A. They are best accessed through a transconjunctival incision
    B. They are best assessed by asking the patent to look upwards
    C. They are part of the middle lamella of the eyelid
    D. Retrobulbar bleeding most commonly occurs from the temporal pad
    E. The inferior oblique muscle separates the medial from the central fat pad

13. **Which of the following is most common following microdermabrasion of the face?**
    A. Hyperpigmentation
    B. Telangiectasia
    C. Bruising
    D. Scarring
    E. Herpes simplex reactivation

14. **A 24-year-old patient presents with a discrete flat patch of purple skin with well-defined borders which has been present from birth. Which wavelength of laser is most effective for cosmetic improvements of its appearance?**

    A. 585 nm
    B. 694 nm
    C. 1,064 nm
    D. 2,940 nm
    E. 10,600 nm

15. **A patient is 4 hours post-bilateral otoplasty utilizing a Mustardé technique. They are experiencing persistent pain from one ear. The best intervention on the ward would be:**

    A. Suction
    B. Compression bandage
    C. Release of all sutures
    D. Injection of local anaesthesia
    E. Intravenous antibiotics

1. B. Open roof deformity. Dorsal hump reduction leaves a flattened dorsum (the 'open roof' deformity) unless lateral osteotomies are completed to in-fracture and correct this. Spreader grafts may be warranted to mitigate against internal nasal valve collapse and breathing difficulties subsequent to this manoeuvre.

2. E. Cephalic trim of the lower lateral cartilages. This question plays on a working knowledge of approaches. In the closed approach there is really little in the way of tip work that can be done, but in the 'delivery' method closed approach the lower lateral cartilages can be 'delivered' to enable cephalic trimming. Remember, you cannot access the tip by definition if you are doing a closed approach.

3. B. Greater auricular nerve. The nerve is easily injured in raising the flap and plicated the platysma and SMAS and is the commonest complication in terms of nerve injury for this procedure, with the marginal mandibular nerve being the next most commonly injured.

4. C. Nanofat grafting. The key is in the detail. This has to be a superficial injection technique for static rhytids, so the choices are between nanofat grafting and fillers. Nanofat is effectively adipocyte-derived adult stem (ADAS) cell transplantation rather than adipocyte grafting, as such having a rejuvenating effect over and above contour correction, which popularizes the technique.

5. A. Scar excision with Z-plasty for reorientation. Simple scar excision will almost certainly lead to recurrence in 100% of cases and is doomed to failure. The other options are all reasonable things to attempt in the context of the case presented, often in combination with each other.

6. B. Acyclovir. Patients with previous history of herpes infections require prophylactic administration of acyclovir, as chemical peels are liable to reactivate the virus.

7. C. Direct brow lift. For a patient who is advanced age with multiple co-morbidities, a direct brow lift can easily be done under local anaesthetic in the outpatients setting and provides a good static repair that will enable him to see on upgaze during his snooker game.

8. A. Alar batten grafts. Only alar batten grafts from the suggested option will support the lower third of the nose and aim to correct external valve collapse.

9. B. Platysma. This can be done as a regional pedicled transfer and provides similar muscle strength with easily 'learnt' movements to simulate a more natural and dynamic smile in the correction of facial asymmetry. In this question, the masseter is the 'distractor question'.

10. B. Fasanella–Servat tarso-mullerectomy. The correct choice of surgical technique depends on an accurate determination of the degree of ptosis and the residual levator function available. In the situation presented here, a limited resection is performed of the conjunctiva, Muller's muscle, and superior third of the tarsal plate. The remaining options are all more aggressive techniques, besides the Kuhnt–Szymanowski procedure, which is a technique employed in ectropion correction. We debated about leaving this question in as there seems to be a move away from eponymous techniques; however, some remain in the examination and we felt it would force the reader to learn about ptosis correction, which is poorly understood by our maxillofacial surgery peers. There are a number of different procedures based on degree of ptosis and residual function.

11. C. Mid-dermal. In this level of burn, a patient will still have sensation but slow capillary refill. Their skin will be darkened pink and will likely have large blisters.

12. D. Retrobulbar bleeding most commonly occurs from the temporal pad. In the lower lids, there are three fat pads: medial, central, and temporal. The medial fat pad is the most vascular and most likely to cause a post-operative retrobulbar bleed following removal in blepharoplasty. If lid skin +/− muscle removal is required, a subconjunctival approach is not appropriate.

13. B. Telangiectasia. Post-operative telangiectasia is the most common side effect of microdermabrasion of the face, especially in thinner skin subtypes. Post-inflammatory hyperpigmentation and scarring generally only occurs in overly aggressive technique due to breaks in the skin. Herpes simplex reactivation after microdermabrasion around the lips is actually very rare.

14. A. 585 nm. This patient most likely has a port-wine stain representing a capillary vascular malformation. Pulsed dye lasers produce pulses of visible light at a wavelength of 585 or 595 nm, with pulse durations of the order of 0.45–40 ms. This wavelength specifically targets oxyhaemoglobin and is the laser of choice for this particular vascular malformation. The remaining wavelengths in this question are commonly used lasers for other head and neck pathology: 694 nm (Q-switched ruby), 1,064 nm (Q-switched neodymium:yttrium-aluminium-garnet), 2,940 nm (erbium), and 10,600 nm (carbon dioxide).

15. A. Suction. Sudden-onset, persistent, or unilateral pain should raise the index of suspicion for haematoma. The dressings should be removed and the area examined for fluctuance. If suspected, the area should be anaesthetized with local anaesthetic, and the minimal number of sutures removed directly over the maximum convexity to enable suction of the haematoma. The haematoma should not be squeezed for risk of distorting the reconstruction. A head dressing should be applied, but only mild compression used.

1. **A post-operative oncology patient on the ward is started on bendroflumethiazide. Shortly afterwards they develop abdominal pains, muscle cramps, and increasing irritability. A range of blood tests demonstrates a potassium level of 3.4 mmol/l and a corrected calcium of 2.7 mmol/l. Which of the following is not used in the treatment of this condition?**

   A. Intravenous (IV) fluids
   B. Calcitonin
   C. Bisphosphonates
   D. Vitamin D
   E. Steroids

2. **You are called by the consultant in emergency medicine to see a 4-year-old child with suspected supraglottic obstruction following accidental swallowing of a toy. Oxygen saturation is 92% with supplemental oxygen. Which of the following is not used in the airway management in this scenario?**

   A. Tracheostomy
   B. Cricothyroidotomy
   C. Intubation
   D. Nasopharyngeal airway
   E. Rapid sequence induction

3. **Which of the following statements are true regarding haemophilia and orthognathic surgery?**

   A. Haemophilia is an absolute contraindication for orthognathic surgery
   B. A factor VIII level in the plasma of 50–75% is needed immediately prior to surgery
   C. Factor VII replacement is required in haemophilia A and factor IX replacement in haemophilia B
   D. There is a high risk of hepatitis C virus carriage
   E. Tranexamic acid decreases the amount of factor replacement required

4. **A 40-year-old patient with diabetes presents to the trauma clinic 3 days following a fall. His eye is tense and swollen. Computed tomography (CT) scan from the time of injury demonstrates an orbital floor fracture. C-reactive protein (CRP) is 143. The most appropriate management should be which of the following?**

A. Lateral canthotomy and cantholysis in clinic under local anaesthesia
B. Admission for IV antibiotics following CT scan
C. Admission for IV antibiotics and consent for orbital floor fracture repair
D. Admission for IV antibiotics with blood tests to include creatine
E. Admission for IV antibiotics and consent for surgical debridement

5. **Which of the following is true of consent in young persons?**

A. A person can be presumed to have the capacity to consent after they reach 18 years old
B. The legal framework for the treatment of all children who lack the capacity to consent differs across the UK
C. 13 years old marks the cut-off for when mature children may have the capacity to consent
D. If a child lacks the capacity to consent, you should ask for their parent's consent
E. A parent can override a young person with capacity and consent to treatment that is in their best interests

6. **According to the World Health Organization (WHO) checklist, following a surgical procedure, it is recommended that the scrub nurse verbally confirm all of the following except:**

A. The name of the procedure
B. Whether the procedure was completed as planned
C. Completion of instrument, sponge, and needle counts
D. Specimen labelling
E. Whether there are any equipment problems to be addressed

7. **According to the American Society of Anesthesiologists Physical Status Classification System, which of the following factors pertinent to oral cancer would mean the patient is *not* level II?**

A. Socially drinking alcohol
B. Malnutrition
C. Type 2 diabetes mellitus not requiring insulin
D. Asymptomatic ventricular septal defect
E. Previously treated oral cancer without recurrence

8. **Which of the following is the most powerful analgesic dose?**

A. 100 mg tramadol orally
B. 6 mg morphine intravenously
C. 30 mg morphine orally
D. 60 mg codeine orally
E. 10 mg oxycodone orally

9. You are asked to review a baby on the neonatal unit. The baby has
    profound mandibular hypoplasia and they are struggling with breathing,
    eating, and sleeping. Which of the following is not an appropriate
    treatment option for this baby?

    A. Surgical tracheostomy
    B. Mandibular distraction
    C. Nasogastric feeding
    D. Nasopharyngeal airway
    E. Tongue–lip division

10. You review a patient on the ward who is 8 days post tracheostomy
    insertion as part of a major head and neck cancer case. They have
    a nasogastric tube in situ but have been started on thickened fluids
    yesterday. A chest radiograph demonstrates a right basal infiltrate but
    the patient has good oxygen saturations and is pyrexial. Which of the
    following is true?

    A. Nasogastric feeding should continue until the tracheostomy is removed
    B. This condition may have been affected by the tracheostomy insertion position
    C. The patient should be restarted on antibiotics
    D. The cuff should be inflated until further notice
    E. High-flow oxygen should be instigated for a chemical pneumonitis

1. D. Vitamin D. One of the side effects of a thiazide diuretic is to cause hypokalaemia. Although the potassium is slightly low, it is unlikely to be the cause of symptoms and is managed by oral supplementation. The patient's symptoms are consistent with hypercalcaemia. Vitamin D should not be given in hypercalcaemia as it can worsen it.

2. B. Cricothyroidotomy. An oxygen saturation of 92% with supplemental oxygen suggests rapidly impending respiratory arrest and is an emergency. A surgical airway is rapidly required. A cricothyroidotomy is contraindicated in children as the thyroid cartilage covers the cricothyroid membrane.

3. E. Tranexamic acid decreases the amount of factor replacement required . Adults with haemophilia have one of the highest prevalence rates of hepatitis C virus among all populations at risk for this disease. Patients with haemophilia have successfully undergone bimaxillary orthognathic surgery without complications. A level of factor VIII in the plasma of 50–75% is needed for dentoalveolar surgery, but for procedures such as orthognathic surgery and fracture fixation a plasma level of 75–100% is recommended.

4. D. Admission for IV antibiotics with haematological testing to include creatine. This patient likely has periorbital necrotizing fasciitis. This is a clinical diagnosis and should not wait for a CT scan. The presence of pale-red, tense, and swollen periorbital skin in the setting of a febrile patient with a history of recent injury, as well as leucocytosis and associated tissue emphysema, strongly raises the clinical suspicion. The Laboratory Risk Indicator for Necrotizing Fasciitis (LRINEC) scoring system is used to assist in the identification of necrotizing fasciitis. A score of 6 and above is suggestive of necrotizing fasciitis, for which surgical intervention is indicated. With a CRP of <150, the score will not exceed 5.

5. D. If a child lacks the capacity to consent, you should ask for their parent's consent. According to General Medical Council (GMC) guidance updated April 2018, at 16 a young person can be presumed to have the capacity to consent. A young person under 16 may have the capacity to consent, depending on their maturity and ability to understand what is involved. The legal framework for the treatment of 16- and 17-year-olds who lack the capacity to consent differs across the UK. Parents cannot override the competent consent of a young person to treatment that you consider is in their best interests.

6. B. Whether the procedure was completed as planned. This is false. The WHO checklist recommends that the scrub nurse, surgeon, and anaesthetist identify key concerns for recovery and management of this patient.

7. B. Malnutrition. This is false and is in fact grade 3. A ventricular septal defect is the most common congenital heart defect and if asymptomatic is level II. Socially drinking alcohol is at least grade 2.

8. C. 30 mg morphine orally.   All drugs are compared with morphine as a way of quantifying their analgesic potency. The best approach to this question is to use each medication's conversion factor and express them all in milligrammes of morphine. Tramadol and codeine are 1/10th as strong as morphine. IV morphine is three times as potent as oral. Oxycodone is twice as strong as morphine.

9.   E. Tongue–lip division.   This patient likely has Pierre Robin sequence. Tongue–lip adhesion is performed and not division. In tongue–lip adhesion, the undersurface of the tip of the tongue is sutured to the inside of the lower lip to hold it in a more forward position. If successful, this is released 3–6 months later. This is used more commonly in the United States than the UK.

10.   B. This condition may have been affected by the tracheostomy insertion position.   The Intensive Care Society has produced guidelines entitled 'Standards for the Care of Adult Patients with a Temporary Tracheostomy'. An infiltrate in a dependent lung segment is suggestive of aspiration, when symptoms of a chemical pneumonitis are absent. Symptoms of chemical pneumonitis include sudden shortness of breath and a cough that develops within minutes or hours. Tracheostomy insertion position affects swallowing. The presence of an inflated cuff compresses the oesophagus and makes swallowing difficult for some patients. The presence of an inflated cuff actually makes aspiration more likely.

References

American Society for of Anaesthesiologists Physical Status Classification System. Last Amended on December 13, 2020 Available at: https://www.asahq.org/standards-and-guidelines/asa-physical-status-classification-system

General Medical Council. Decision making and consent. Published 30 September 2020. Available at: https://www.gmc-uk.org/-/media/documents/gmc-guidance-for-doctors---decision-making-and-consent-english_pdf-84191055.pdf

Intensive Care Society. Standards for the Care of Adult Patients with a Temporary Tracheostomy. Published July 2008. Updated on July 2011. Available at: https://icmwk.com/wp-content/uploads/2014/02/care_of_the_adult_patient_with_a_temporary_tracheostomy_2008.pdf

World Health Organisation Surgical Safety Checklist. Revised Jan 2009. Available at: https://www.who.int/teams/integrated-health-services/patient-safety/research/safe-surgery/tool-and-resources

1. **Which one of these statistical measures is least affected by outliers?**
    A. Mean
    B. Median
    C. Standard deviation
    D. Range
    E. Mode

2. **You are reading a study about quality of life immediately after surgery for oral cancer. In which type of study does 'recall bias' pose a substantial problem?**
    A. Retrospective case-controlled study
    B. Prospective study cohort study
    C. Meta-analysis
    D. Crossover study
    E. Randomized double blind study

3. **A study demonstrates that the combined odds ratio for tobacco smoking related to oral cancer was 4.65, with a 95% confidence interval of 0.54–0.93. Which of the following is true?**
    A. 2.5% of measured values will lie below the lower limit of the interval
    B. 95% of the measured values will lie within the limits of the interval
    C. 5% of sample means will lie above the upper limit of the interval
    D. There is a 5% chance of the population mean lying above the upper limit of the interval
    E. The population mean lies within the limits of the interval with 95% confidence

4. **The relative risk for oral cancer is 5.3 for people who smoke less than 15 cigarettes per day. Regarding this relative risk, which of the following is true?**
    A. It is the probability of an event occurring in smokers relative to non- smokers
    B. It can be positive or negative
    C. It describes the chance of a patient's family developing oral cancer
    D. It is calculated by the square root of the mean incidence in the smoking group divided by the mean incidence in the non-smoking group
    E. When the risk is equal amongst the exposed and unexposed group, the value is 0

5. What is the best design of study to assess the incidence of leukoplakia in patients who smoke presenting to an oral and maxillofacial surgery department?

A. Case controlled

B. Cohort

C. Cross sectional

D. Qualitative

E. Randomized controlled trial

1. E. Mode. The mode is the value least affected by outliers, followed by the median and the interquartile range. The mean in particular shows significant change with outliers, such as increasing with a high outlier.

2. A. Retrospective case-controlled study. Recall bias is of particular concern in retrospective studies that use a case-control design to investigate the aetiology of a disease. This can potentially exaggerate the relation between a potential risk factor and the disease.

3. E. The population mean lies within the limits of the interval with 95% confidence. A 95% confidence interval is a range of values that you can be 95% certain contains the true mean of the population. Crucially it is not the same as a range that contains 95% of the values.

4. A. It is the probability of an event occurring in smokers relative to non-smokers. In this case the relative risk combines the risk of oral cancer in smokers versus non-smokers. However, care must be taken, in that the underlying absolute risks are concealed and readers tend to overestimate the effect when it is presented in relative terms.

5. B. Cohort. In a cohort study, a group of individuals exposed to a putative risk factor and a group who are unexposed to the risk factor are followed over time to determine the occurrence of disease. The incidence of disease in the exposed group is compared with the incidence of disease in the unexposed group.

INDEX